Behavioural and Social
Rehabilitation and Training

Behavioural and Social Rehabilitation and Training

Roy I. Brown and **E. Anne Hughson**

Rehabilitation Studies Programme
Faculty of Education
The University of Calgary

JOHN WILEY & SONS
Chichester · New York · Brisbane · Toronto · Singapore

Copyright © 1987 by John Wiley & Sons Ltd.

Library of Congress Cataloging-in-Publication Data:

Brown, Roy I.
  Behavioural and social rehabilitation and training.

  Includes index.
  1. Rehabilitation. I. Hughson, E. Anne. II. Title.
[DNLM: 1. Handicapped. 2. Mental Retardation—rehabilitation. WM 308 B879b]
RM930.B75 1987   617   86−28952

ISBN 0 471 91149 6

British Library Cataloguing in Publication Data:

Brown, Roy I.
  Behavioural and social rehabilitation and training.
  1. Rehabilitation
  I. Title II. Hughson, E. Anne
  362.4′048   RM930

ISBN 0 471 91149 6

Typeset by Woodfield Graphics, Arundel, West Sussex.

Printed and bound in Great Britain by Anchor Brendon Ltd, Essex.

*This book is dedicated
to our families*

Contents

Preface

This book has been developed as a result of experience in a wide range of demonstration research and clinical situations. During this time we have become concerned about the large accumulation of data concerning disabled persons, particularly mentally handicapped persons, and the lack of attempts to pull these data together into some sort of model or models. Students commencing to read this material during their undergraduate or graduate programmes would, in fact, never have finished by the time they were thought ready to practise in the field or retire! Many professionals have commented on the increase in the research-to-practice gap, and it seems to us that one of the effective ways of reducing this is to ensure that the practitioner has a series of guidelines or principles to apply within the rehabilitation field. In particular we are referring to the rehabilitation education field with its particular interest in behaviour, social issues and competence training. Such a task is an arduous one and fraught with a wide range of problems. We are very much aware of the dangers of over-simplification, and of glossing over contradictory evidence, but despite this we believe that such an attempt at model-building would be worthwhile for ourselves, and for other colleagues who wish to practise in the broad field of rehabilitation education. It will become apparent that we believe the field must necessarily be transdisciplinary, and therefore knowledge from a wide range of areas needs to be employed.

Our aim is to attempt to bring research and practice together and provide practitioners with a set of guidelines or principles which will help them and their clients in practice. We encourage the reader to be critical of these principles and not to see them as watertight statements. Wherever possible we have given practical examples. Our evidence is from both the clinical and research fields.

It has been recognized for some while that any one set of processes may not solve a specific learning problem. The field requires a range of problem-solving strategies which can be applied in a consistent manner in order to build effective interventions for any one individual. It is with these ideas in mind that the following chapters have been written. It is hoped that in generating some more comprehensive model we may encourage a closer look at the broader concepts of training, education and rehabilitation as they apply to specific individuals, and as they apply to society at large.

In the following chapters several specific areas are discussed in relation to a rehabilitation model. One aspect concerns the development of training continua in the programme service delivery areas. It should be recognized that this is an external systematic structuring of the sequence and methods of training skills with a view to providing a technology for the delivery of programmes in an interactive and holistic manner. This is in many ways artificial, and it must be recognized that this part of the model should be applied in a general fashion and not be imposed arbitrarily in any specific manner. It sets a framework in which to examine the services involved in rehabilitation education. The model is intended as a a guide to structuring information about training for application by a wide range of rehabilitation practitioners. It also is a means by which expertise in teaching adaptive skills can be delivered, not just to people with one handicapping condition, but to people with a wide range of differing disabilities. Hopefully, it provides a structured guide for assessing the learning processes and needs of the individual in order to direct the particular education or training required.

Another section of the book applies a wide range of behavioural phenomena, which seem to be important in understanding how individuals function. It attempts to harness known training strategies and tactics within a comprehensive model of rehabilitation. This particular section emphasizes that individuals with disabilities are neither static nor are they continuous in their growth processes; that is, skills are gained and lost. The reasons for gain or losss relate to the stresses and strains within the individuals and their environments. One major aspect of this oscillation of behaviour relates to ecological structures, and these have to be interpreted and taken into account in setting up individual behavioural plans for each individual. A third section examines the implication of the guidelines for assessment and programme practice.

A further section attempts to apply a model to the service delivery concerns of staff education and management. It is argued that management structures are affected by the same types of phenomena that are described in the previous sections; that is, there needs to be some external structuring of the management system of any agency or service that is delivered, and this must relate to the behavioural needs of clients and staff. Staff gain, organize and apply knowledge, within a particular system which is itself subject to behavioural cycles of regression and growth. It is the total integration of the systems which must be appreciated if we are to develop effective services for people with a broad range of developmental and other disabilities. The section is followed by an examination of the roles of advocacy and self-advocacy as they affect the rehabilitation process, and the relevance of the preceding chapters to professional staff development.

In bringing together our material we have decided to explore the relationship between what might be termed rehabilitation education and some of the more recent knowledge in brain activity. Here we are aware that speculation may have its dangers, and that the examination of the microstructures within the central nervous system is at an early stage of development. Our arguments in this field should therefore be taken extremely cautiously. Yet we do see a parallel between what is occurring in terms of behaviour and some of the knowledge that has been generated within the psychoneurological field.

In developing this book we gratefully acknowledge the advice, comment and assistance of a number of people. First of all, our students have been asked to comment on the principles as we have developed them or culled them from the literature. Many of them seem to have found the process a useful one, and have made many suggestions which they have derived from the type of model put forward. Thus we feel the method is an important one from a didactic point of view. In particular Sister Maureen O'Connell was helpful in writing a written commentary on some of the earlier drafts of chapters. We would like to acknowledge the input of Professor Peter Mittler, who critically evaluated a draft of the material. His detailed comments have been very helpful to us, and wherever possible we have tried to make use of his suggestions. Obviously the final version, with its pros and cons, is our responsibility, and we offer it as a start in the development of models of rehabilitation. We would also like to thank Mary Brown for suggesting ways that we might simplify the material, or display it more effectively, and for carrying out detailed proof reading.

We would like to thank Linda Culshaw for typing the various drafts, and Elizabeth Brown for artwork in developing the figures. We would also like to thank our publisher, Mr Michael Coombs, who patiently waited for various drafts and provided advice and encouragement as we slowly progressed towards the final version.

RIB
EAH
1986

CHAPTER ONE

An overview to rehabilitation

Introduction

This book is about rehabilitation and it presents, admittedly, a particular view; a view which has been developed from demonstration, research and practice in the field. It concerns primarily the psychological, social and educational aspects of rehabilitating individuals into the community.

Society has gradually changed its ideas about the nature of ability in people with disabling conditions, and it is believed now that neither genetics nor environmental knowledge alone explains their behaviour. Nor can we forecast results of treatment for any individual or programme with any degree of accuracy (Clarke and Clarke, 1974; Wortis, 1981). Research workers have, over a 30-year period, carried out a range of experiments and observations, and in a variety of ways influenced the rehabilitation scene. We now possess new knowledge and new ideas; yet if one looks at the voluminous range of research articles, for example in the volumes relating to the Scientific Study of Mental Deficiency (Berg, 1982), certain basic problems emerge.

Setting the scene—work programmes

Since the Second World War a vast amount of information—including experimental data and demonstration and practice from training centres, schools and hospitals—has been made available. Despite this, or perhaps because of it, research workers and training staff have become concerned that there is a gap between research and practice. A variety of articles (Clarke, 1977; Mittler, 1977) detail some of these concerns. However, this research—practice gap remains, and may be increasing (Brown, 1981a). The thesis of this book is that this divergence results largely from the lack of a comprehensive model of rehabilitation from which to interpret the work. Without this we are distracted from building new processes from which new techniques, programmes and relevant questions can be developed. Or perhaps we have now developed enough history to restructure the disparate aspects of rehabilitation into a theory that can generate a working model.

During the late 1940s the development of the first training workshops for persons with mental handicaps occurred in Britain under an experimental or research model.

The model was largely one of vocational output and work rather than any more broad-based model of rehabilitation. It was apparent, with the inclusion of many mentally handicapped people in the war effort, that it might well be possible to train individuals in skills of a vocational nature. It was out of necessity, and experience in that necessity, that new ideas developed. It is suggested that this was a sensible place to start, possibly the only place to start, for man's knowledge tends to develop from the concrete to the abstract. More recently home living skills and even leisure time skills have been viewed as important aspects of training. Yet we are still largely in a vocational mode in terms of adult rehabilitation.

In North America a similar movement occurred whereby adult developmentally handicapped individuals were placed into vocational settings. This seemed to be part of the general parent movement that had maintained their children when younger within the community and now were looking for options when they were too old for school. Similar to the segregated school concept, the vocational services were developed as a day activity programme, still segregated, but allowing individuals to have something to do during the day. This thrust to plan vocationally for young adults began in the late 1950s and early 1960s, and it, too, was concerned more with work output and 'being actively at work' rather than in a broader-based model of rehabilitation.

Over the past years the notion of vocational rehabilitation and sheltered workshops has developed and, at its best, vocational training is seen as a broader goal for training social competence than the work activity programmes generally referred to as sheltered workshops. However it has become common practice to assume that vocational learning is the most important type of adult learning, and that this is the vehicle for adult rehabilitation. It is true that a wide range of group opportunities have developed for home living, but these are insufficient and cater for a relatively small group of people. It should be noted that most disabled adults receive vocational training in day programmes while returning to their own homes at night. Integrated programming is relatively rare (e.g. in Ontario one programme in a large urban area offers day training to over 300 people, of whom 82 per cent do not receive home living training).

Development of social and allied skill training

Traditionally professionals providing vocational training programmes do not intervene within the individual's home. This is particularly true of the older adult who may remain with his parents throughout his life. The need for social skill learning, leisure time learning and home living skill learning has not been clearly understood; yet, as we shall see later, it is probably amongst these environments that the most abstract and more necessary training should occur. It is argued, therefore, that in putting forward our concepts of rehabilitation we must consider the wide range of lifestyles which confront the particular individual. Data suggest that many mentally handicapped people fail in the 'outside' world after they have been through vocational training because they run into problems associated with other aspects of their lifestyle. It will be noted that the precipitating cause may not be in the vocational area or an inability to do one's work, but rather in an inability to deal with some of the problems of home living or allied skills. For example, issues relating to recreational and leisure time activities may be of considerable importance in this context.

Concrete and abstract levels of programming

It is argued that within the programme areas the more abstract and the more diverse the overall training content, the more critical it becomes to maintain the individual effectively within the community. As we become more aware of the skills essential to surviving in our communities we must recognize the limitations in our knowledge of how to apply the research in learning to 'real-life' situations. Much of our measurement over the past years has been in observable, concretely measured units, for example, number of 'widgets' produced per hour. The more covert and abstract processes associated with thought, motivation and self-image are only now coming under closer scrutiny. However, it is these which will be essential in the development of future rehabilitation programmes. The work of individuals such as Feuerstein (1979), who have looked at the process of mediated learning, provides good examples of these internal processes. Also Rosen, Clark and Kivitz's (1977) observations of social motivation and self-image as important components in the learning process are essential to building a more comprehensive model.

Research, experimentation and practice

Probably at no other time in our history have we found it more necessary to collaborate across the sciences, and to recognize that it is through transdisciplinary involvement (Brown, 1984b) that understanding of rehabilitation procedures may be furthered. Yet, in its own way, this is a new fumbling in the dark, for we have only old structures and untried abilities with which to construct new structures, to explain, define or redirect our future endeavours.

In this technical age it is often felt that experimentation will provide the answer to our questions. It becomes more and more apparent that creative ideas are divorced from the process of experimentation (Marlett, 1986). Experimentation is the technical means whereby we attempt to estimate the veracity of ideas, and it is unlikely that experimentation will amount to much unless we are able to produce meaningful ideas which are understood by our society. The problem has always been where to start for, in the jigsaw, it is impossible in the beginning to know which pieces go together when we have no idea of what the picture is. Unless we are willing to take the pieces that have been identified and attempt to formulate them into some plan or model for understanding or conceptualizing our picture, it is unlikely that we will be able to test new ideas or devise new techniques and processes.

For some while we have, reasonably, been concerned with the measurement of abilities in man, and have devised a range of tests to assess these abilities (Anastasi, 1968; Mittler, 1970). We have become aware of the notion of error and recognize that the results we obtain may be fallible, not predicting later development nor validly measuring what we think we are measuring (Clarke, Clarke and Brown, 1956). It is a fatal mistake to deny the importance of this stage of development. It appears throughout the history of man that one stage logically precedes the development of another, and the second stage cannot exist without its forerunner. Thus the initial stages must have their place in history, and it is dangerous to suppose that, by the denial of earlier periods or the rewriting of history, we will find new truths ahead of us. Such is the case in the matter of the denial of measurement of ability in terms of its use in society. It may be true that intelligence tests are not appropriate measures of performance in predicting future accomplishments of children with mental handicaps (Stott, 1977). This does not deny the place that tests have had in understanding human abilities. Nor does it assert that these tests are in their final form, for they must develop into more sophisticated measures which can provide new and more reliable data.

Much of the literature in behavioural science, and more specifically in the behavioural studies of mental handicap in the 1950s and 1960s, was of an experimental nature; that is, research workers attempted to apply the process of experimental methodology to the field of psychology, believing that it would tease out and provide answers to a range of questions.

Over this time some researchers and practitioners have come to believe that psychology cannot be viewed at this stage as primarily an experimental science, and others that research is more appropriately placed at an ethological or observational level where individual behaviour is examined in natural situations (Sluckin, 1964; Hutt, Hutt and Ounstead, 1965; Edgerton, 1967).

The process of error and intragroup variability

In attempting to understand the process of rehabilitation it is necessary to recognize that we live in a changing society, and that the natures of psychological argument and psychological data are to some degree ephemeral and may relate only to particular events, at particular points in time. The process that works today may not have worked yesterday, and may not work tomorrow. It is not the technique which will necessarily last, but more likely the principles and processes that underlie behavioural change. It is fashionable to decry what has been carried out by our predecessors. It is certainly true that in their honest, and sometimes dishonest, gropings towards the truth, they have at times put aside the most important items of information. One example of this relates to that which many scientists have come to regard as artifacts or trends in data which they believe represent statistical wastage. It just may be that this error contains the fundamental seeds of explanation for much of our behaviour.

In the field of rehabilitation it has become obvious that variability in human functioning is closely related to concepts of treatment and programming, and this variability represents some of the most important information in terms of understanding how clients respond. Programming of behaviour, in terms of change, must be related to baseline performance. Behaviour, and indeed experimentation, appear at this point of time to be based largely on the idea of group examination. Our newsprint is full of examples of the effects of this or that drug, or one food or another, on longevity, on illnesses and on mental health. What is interesting about such studies is that they are often contradicted, within a fairly short period of time, by other studies showing that the item which was supposed to be most disastrous to our health in fact is of essential need for some other group of people. For example there are studies involving cholesterol, suggesting that it is harmful in terms of an individual's longevity, but this is contradicted by other studies suggesting that people who do not have cholesterol in sufficient amounts are likely to die rather early. It is claimed that certain food additives cause distractibility, attention disruption, and hyperactivity (Kinsbourne and Caplan, 1979), while other studies show little or no effects due to drug or food additives (Johnson and Morasky, 1977). The fact of the matter is that the intragroup variability in many studies is greater than the intergroup variability, but this only suggests that we are probably not measuring the appropriate variables or setting up the necessary contrast groups. Some individuals may be affected at some time by certain conditions, because the general level of environmental stimulation and their internal states make them vulnerable at that particular point.

Individual performance

Although a number of workers have pointed to intragroup and intergroup variability (Gunzburg, 1968; Mittler, 1981), it seems quite clear that the health services generally, and psychology in particular, have not paid sufficient attention to the individual's own performance variance. As far back as 1956, Bartlett and Shapiro suggested, in the field of learning disability, that individual studies of the performance of children were important, and that experimental models could be developed for examining an individual's specific behaviours. This approach has never had a very large following within the field of psychology. However, it is now being recognized in the educational field that individual programme planning, baseline assessment, and the provision of particular programmes for specific individuals are all important. It is of interest that this has arisen out of two considerations: one the range of scientific methodology and experimentation from the late 1950s onwards, and the other the large and vigorous response from parents (Sarason and Doris, 1979) concerned about the lack of suitable accommodation or conditions of education for their children.

What should be of interest to the behavioural scientist are the results on some measures of individual variability, and yet in many of the early studies, where analysis was possible, authors have ignored these results. Another example of researchers' exclusion or misinterpretation of their own data is given by Carol Gilligan (1982) in her review of the sociological work regarding moral structure and development in relation to gender difference. Her reviews of the data collected for female subjects, in tests of moral and ethical development, suggest that unexplained variability was thrown out rather than interpreted within the overall model of emotional development.

Perhaps it is important to stress that the immediate post-Second World War studies, particularly in the growing professional field of psychology, dealt with highly formal laboratory experimentation using large groups of subjects. Gradually the research moved to vocational training environments for handicapped people (e.g. Clarke and Hermelin, 1955; O'Connor and Tizard, 1956). Other workers, such as Woodward (1960), looked at handicapped children's play and problem-solving behaviour. Gradually this more natural environment for experimentation led to (a) the need to respond to individual difference; (b) a more humanitarian concern with handicapped individuals as people, particularly as rehabilitation was undertaken; and (c) an awareness by parents that change and development was possible and all was not 'lost' for their children.

Assessment in rehabilitation

It has been apparent for some time that intelligence is a poor predictor of overall life skills performance in persons with mental handicap, and that many people with low intelligence do as well as, if not better than, people with higher intelligence. Cobb (1972), in reviewing over 200 studies, confirms this view, yet intelligence tests are still employed to predict certain aspects of performance. Some recent work (McKerracher et al., 1980) suggests that certain aspects of adult living or function-ing may be associated with measured intelligence, while other areas may not. It is interesting, for example, that intelligence measures appear to be correlated with educational attainment when predicting specific educational skills, but not necess-arily associated with social skills attainment. If one develops a socially oriented curriculum, then intelligence does not seem to be as relevant to prediction of success. It therefore becomes very important to recognize what the teaching goals are, and what expectations are contained within any particular curriculum. It is not sufficient for educators to demand more practical social training unless clarification between a social curriculum and a formal academic curriculum has been addressed.

Much more important than this, however, is the concept that social skills, which are apparently not closely related to intelligence measures (McKerracher et al., 1980), might be far more important in terms of whether an individual can or cannot survive in society. For years there has been the argument concerning the use of intel-ligence testing within the rehabilitation process. Many psychologists, and certainly other professionals, require such data, and one suspects that it provides them with some type of marker which supports other findings. It could also be used as a base-line for interpreting certain specific difficulties. Unfortunately these test results are often used as an administrative tool, not only to designate people under particular labels, but to restrict the environments in which people live, work or learn. Recent data suggest an answer to the dilemma of whether intelligence is relevant or not in the area of mental handicap. The work of Halpern and Fuhrer (1984), Brown, Bayer and MacFarlane (1986), and Wehman (1981) in the area of functional assessment and curriculum development may have a far greater impact on programme delivery and planning than the previous emphasis on the interpretation and recommendation arising from cognitive tests of performance. The development of functional assess-ment tests to determine needs and strengths of persons with chronic mental illness has also generated new dimensions to community rehabilitation. Obviously the results of these directions have led to new optimism about successful reintegration into community life.

For a long period of time it had been assumed that mentally handicapped people needed the same type of programme as normal youngsters. The work of Earl (1961), followed by that of Gunzburg (1968), illustrated fairly clearly that other types of skills were important in the development of handicapped youngsters. The development of tests such as the Progress Assessment Chart (PAC) (Gunzburg, 1969)— which attempted to measure some of the basic elements of vocational, occupational and allied skills, including communication and social and educational skills—were seen as important. Later other techniques such as the Adaptive Functioning Index (Marlett, 1971) were developed. Tests measuring social educational skills, rather than formal academic requirements, included concepts relating to what individuals needed to know to perform, and likewise the distinction between whether they had opportunities to perform various items or were unable to perform them was recognized. Such concepts were related to vocational, residential and social performance.

Normalization

The observation that disabled individuals can be rehabilitated into society has gradually led us to put forward concepts of normalization (Grunewald, 1969; Nirje, 1970; Wolfensberger, 1972) and more recently to argue, in many of our communities, for the integration of handicapped youngsters into regular school classes. Much of this has not been based on an experimental approach to education or psychology, or social welfare. Some of it has resulted from individual experience, out of humanitarian need, and in many places has become associated with an ideology that has led to the approach of social change agentry. This may be doomed to die or metamorphose as new motivations, causes, and preachers develop in our communities. Social change and societal shifts in attitudes were very much a part of the 1960s and early 1970s. Minority groups and those who were still oppressed (e.g. women, black people) were beginning to speak out in society. In many ways more humanitarian concerns for disabled and handicapped persons were occurring in the same societal context. In other words North American society in particular was ripe for such changes in attitude towards people who were perceived as deviant.

First starting in Sweden and other Scandinavian countries, normalization has been expanded in North America through the work of people such as Wolfensberger (1972). The theme, simply stated, is one in which handicapped individuals are helped and encouraged to grow, and participate in life, as far as they can, on a normal basis. Wolfensberger (1983) has furthered his definition by describing 'normal' as 'culturally valued' and renaming normalization as 'social role valorization'. In doing this, few have troubled to consider what is normal or valued; nor have they imagined the changing nature of our society which, suitable perhaps for an individual at one stage of his growth, is no longer suitable several years later when society has changed its systems, its techniques or its attitudes towards handicapped individuals.

Normalization is a philosophy, and one which many of us espouse. Yet its major weakness in the form in which it is accepted in North America acts as a major drawback to many of the plans developed for handicapped people. It is a philosophy without an accepted technology, and more importantly neither philosophy nor technology are built into any form of model. Without a model from which to build, it is unlikely that we will develop the type of staff or the programmes which can bring about normalization. The development of new programmes has essentially involved exposing people to stimulation rather than training people how to deal with stimulation (Gold, 1973). It has been done by dumping people suddenly in the community and pretending that this is normalization. The major losers in such a procedure are handicapped people themselves, for it will be quickly said that normalization has been tried and has failed, and the failure is because people with handicaps do not have sufficient ability.

There are possibly several critical explanations as to why the application of normalization is faltering within our communities. One important consideration may be that society does not really understand or desire to design programmes or spend money in natural community settings. It may not be part of society's general belief system that handicapped people can gradually learn how to adapt. Therefore we become quick to say that normalization has failed because the work is too difficult and too expensive. Furthermore, the political decision-makers are not willing to take up that challenge for change. In addition society has not developed programmes to provide adequately skilled staff to teach handicapped youngsters. Slow learning means what it says, and individuals are not likely to change by merely presenting them with reasonable conditions, however appropriate these may be in their own right. It is the development of programme strategies which can enable people gradually to increase their learning power and thus their adaptation to society. Once again this relates not just to the field of mental handicap, but to all specialized groups who are segregated from society or are treated as aberrant within society. A major example in Canada today is the large number of homeless and unemployed people in urban areas where many of the issues of self-image and stress are similar to those in specific rehabilitation fields (Holosko, 1987).

Generalization of findings

During this time of change a wealth of new data has become available, and it seems an appropriate time to attempt to formulate such data into some model or models of rehabilitation. It would seem, too, that the models of rehabilitation may have wider applicability than simply a resolution of the problems of mental handicap, and are relevant to a range of individuals who have problems in adaptation in our society for a variety of reasons. Indeed one could argue that the formulations go much further than this, and apply to our society as a whole. It is intriguing to contemplate how often specific information has a wider general applicability than its original purpose. We only have to look at examples in the space industry to recognize the larger benefits to mankind in the areas of engineering, construction and medical science.

The same process can work the other way, for it seems obvious that some of the techniques developed in rehabilitation have relevance to general behaviour in society. This book attempts to put together a range of information and to explain a range of behaviours that suggest a model for future exploration. It is not suggested that it is a complete model; nor does it pretend that it is entirely based on data, whether that be experimental or observational. It also attempts to generalize specific behavioural results, a process often condemned by the experimental behaviourist, who is concerned that this results in scientific error. This is acknowledged. Yet ideas are the substance of exploration and the motivators of proper experimentation. It is for the reader to judge whether the ideas expressed here have any relevance to that particular process. There is also, in the field of rehabilitation, a growing recognition that the study of individual cases provides example and detail that demonstrates knowledge across individual need and variability (Sarason and Doris, 1979).

Major studies concerning growth

Normalization assumes growth and change. Although earlier researchers (Itard, 1801; Seguin, 1846; Binet and Simon, 1916) recognized the possibilities of growth and change, much of the early twentieth century saw scientists and educators perceiving a model which accepted the constancy of cognitive ability (Clarke and Clarke, 1954). But in the 1950s and 1960s it gradually became accepted that cognitive functioning is not static within an individual. Individuals show considerable increase in capabilities at various times in their lives (Honzik, MacFarlane and Allen, 1948). Where this concerns a mentally handicapped person from an adverse environment it is known that he or she is likely to show large increases in cognitive functioning during the late teens and twenties. It is apparent from the work of Vernon (1951) that individuals who, as adults, work in skilled rather than unskilled professions, maintain their functioning level in terms of cognitive ability unlike their unskilled counterparts. It is also believed that early intervention shows major effects on performance (Bronfenbrenner, 1976). Young children subjected to early stimulation, which is environmentally enriched, appear to show considerable increase in growth rates (e.g. Heber and Garber, 1971; Lazar and Darlington, 1978). Yet such early intervention must be continued if it is to have a lasting effect (Bricker, Seibert and Casuso, 1980).

Overall there are a number of facts which suggest some of the variables involved in effecting the magnitude of environmental damage. Early damage or adversity appears to have a profound effect upon growth, and it has been suggested by some that this may delay early growth spurts during the first five or six years of life. Clarke and Clarke (1959) have suggested that secondary growth spurts may occur during the late teens and early twenties. It seems possible that attention processes are damaged by early institutionalization or adversity of environment (Robinson and Robinson, 1965). It is apparent that increased parental involvement, parental stimulation and knowledge all seem to diffuse the effects of retardation. Bronfenbrenner (1976) has itemized in some detail the major impacts of early intervention and long-term stimulation which appear to be necessary if growth is going to not only occur, but be maintained. Similar issues and comment are discussed by Bromwich (1981) in relation to high-risk mothers and children. These all speak to the idea that intervention is a complex and long-term process.

Rehabilitation models

This book is about rehabilitation, and a concern that the types of models which enable society to provide a highly sophisticated and professional service have not yet been developed. This is not to deny the work that has been done by a vast range of professionals, nor to underestimate the contributions that have been made in the past. There is a need to examine societal developments as well as the knowledge that exists within specific sciences, together with current rehabilitation practice, in order to come forward with models which can assist not only in enhancing service, but also in improving the thrusts of research and application, which we believe are required in the short as well as the long term. In doing this we are aware that we will raise some eyebrows, and that experimenters and practitioners alike may find some of their vested interests questioned. It should be recognized that an attempt is being made to integrate findings and experience, some of it clinical, some of it experimental, and some of it based on the broader views of society and human functioning.

It is probably a truism to state that society develops processes as it requires them. Man is an ambivalent animal who on the one hand shows curiosity about his environment, and on the other hand is sufficiently practical so that he only builds structures as he requires them. In the post-Freudian era, man has become increasingly concerned about the behavioural processes which direct his living, and has come to recognize that many of his responses are governed by a range of variables, which interact with one another, and culminate in behaviour which is generically recognized as personality. Although we have not developed the tools to measure or interpret behavioural responses adequately, it is essentially during the last half of the twentieth century that a variety of new tools have been explored which may possibly help in an understanding of the intricacies of our own behaviour. Some of these tools relate to the measurement of environment (Wolfensberger and Glenn, 1975) for it is recognized that behaviour is frequently contingent on the environment in which it occurs. The commencement of such analysis of environment is seen in the writings of Cantrell and Cantrell (1980), and the description of ecology described in the 'meso, exo and macro systems' offered by Bronfenbrenner (1979), and more recently by Mitchell (1986). Interestingly, an integrated environmental and behavioural assessment technique does not appear to have been produced.

An integrated model

The thesis of this book is that rehabilitation, to be effective, must be based on an integrated model which touches all aspects of life of the disabled individual. But such a model might well apply to the lives of other people such as those with a mental illness, certain elderly persons, or accident victims, who so often are medically treated, but then face a long road of social and psychological adjustment before they can fully enter, or reasonably enter, normal society. This general application, which appears to cut across age groups (Brown, 1984b), makes it unnecessary to separate habilitation from rehabilitation or regard different disability groups as having different learning processes. Regardless of disability there are social requirements, expectations and performance criteria which are held in common.

The case made in this book is that with a model we can apply some general rules and procedures to all the rehabilitative fields, and put forward new strategies which will help to overcome some of the difficulties outlined. In one sense the theoretical views expressed in this book might not be those which are accepted by the pure experimental investigator. It is not claimed that they necessarily explain all the facts that are available to us. Rather, it attempts to integrate some of our knowledge and produce a coherent integration of that knowledge from which more appropriate models may be developed. It must be recognized that working with individuals with a developmental handicap is an extremely skilled occupation. It is one where care and concern are indeed appropriate, but without in-depth knowledge of training strategies little improvement is likely to occur in the majority of cases.

General conceptualization

It is also the thesis of this book that the principles in the rehabilitation process are not extraordinary ones in terms of their application to human functioning. In other words, any coherent system which is developed should be relevant to all individuals, not merely to some subsection of the population.

The problem at the present time is that when research workers develop new processes their findings are often not integrated into the practical field. Worse than this, where there have been attempts to blend research and practice, we find that once research workers move on to new aspects of study, the field worker is left isolated once again. Many professionals who come into the field may have techniques, but they rarely have any concept of the philosophy of rehabilitation. Techniques are often not well taught in relation to research and demonstration findings (Paine, Bellamy and Wilcox, 1984). Too often the specifics of research define and replicate concrete behavioural techniques, which are not then integrated into an overall model. Paine et al. (1984) discuss the different issues necessary to field research and demonstration. These include the results of applying behavioural-specific technology versus the demonstration of that technology, and finally, at a more comprehensive level, the integration of the demonstrated methodology into a model. Their criticism is that such models are not put into place, disseminated and evaluated and then integrated into a larger delivery system.

It is suggested that the knowledge gained from studies of child development and handicap, and the research on vocational, social, home living and leisure time programmes for handicapped people, should be integrated and, if possible, bonded together in an overall philosophy and strategy for rehabilitation. This could provide us with a theoretical construct for rehabilitation strategy in the area of environmental programming. Unless such concepts are underpinned in terms of cognitive or central nervous system functioning, it is likely that the model will have only limited applicability. It is suggested that we must now attempt to develop a model where learning interfaces with our knowledge of the central nervous system, and from this develop further models for rehabilitation experimentation.

Research and field workers have for some while criticized the use of organicity and non-organicity as a basis for understanding the origins of behaviour in handicapped persons. A model which employs recent field evidence may suggest that organic versus environmental causation may be a red herring. It seems possible that an integrated theory of rehabilitation may meaningfully support the argument that environmental damage must have specific organic counterparts and therefore represent damage to, or lack of optimum development within, the central nervous system. It is recognized that such an argument is speculative at present and needs to be examined and supported in detail. The matter is taken up further in a later chapter. However, it is an important argument for it may well explain why there is some confusion between the so-called soft signs of organicity and the conflicting statement that they are equally caused by environmental deprivation. In other words, in reality, the organic and environmental arguments are not choices but represent similar viewpoints. Environmental damage which is behavioural may result in organic deficit. If this is true it raises the prospect that control of the central nervous system could take place through the development of environmentally sophisticated learning programmes. The idea, as such, is not new to physiotherapy or occupational therapy which have implicitly, for many years, assumed that by providing adequate external stimulation and manipulation of the body, recovery of various functions would be increased. However this is a far cry from the concept that actually providing appropriate stimulation may facilitate the development of the central nervous system in terms of its structure and biochemistry. In these circumstances brain injury is not seen merely as the result of physical trauma, but as inappropriate delivery of psychological and social stimuli. Our lack of acceptance of this possibility is occasioned not so much by lack of knowledge, but by our inability to conceptualize the role of abstract processes which may be transitory in time. Such processes may be equally as important as the more gross forms of damage which are known to occur. For example, many parents often protect mentally handicapped youngsters from the possibilities of physical damage. This may take place by preventing a young adult riding alone on public transportation, or ensuring that he is always accompanied by someone. Certainly such protective procedures lessen the chances of physical damage. However, they may increase the chances of psychological and social damage. This lack, in its own turn, may result in effective central nervous system damage. Further, the presence of abnormal psychological or social stimulation may occasion the retardation of the central nervous system. This refers to the problems associated with primary and secondary negative impact, for it is often true that the environmental conditions create secondary negative impacts. These are far more subtle in their form than is often recognized, and they are rarely attended to by individuals working in the therapeutic scene.

Advantages and disadvantages of such a model

The disadvantages of attempting to articulate a comprehensive model as outlined above are considerable. First of all it is apparent that there are large gaps in our knowledge, and the development of any model may, in fact, overlook important areas. The data from certain experiments may be falsely generalized to situations in which they do not apply. Worse than this, the development of such a model could indeed cause us to rigidify our thinking and discourage the formulation of experimental work in certain directions. Nevertheless it would seem that the disadvantages are outweighed by a wide range of advantages. The concept of model-building of this type is not new to behavioural science, and in the field of animal behaviour Lorenz (1981) has suggested a model involving a continuum of behaviour. Such models are regarded as 'blueprints', and as such are not rigid or unchangeable since, as in building a structure from a blueprint, many changes are possible (McFarland, 1981). It is essential, as has been pointed out in the ethological context, that rigidity of interpretation can hinder the application or the advance of the science which the model purports to support.

The concept of structure has been introduced. It will be argued that development of a structured approach to learning is essential if handicapped persons are to be rehabilitated. The same process is relevant to our own thinking. Unless we can structure some type of model it becomes difficult to develop our thinking processes further. It may well be that such a model is found wanting, and certainly will be replaced as new evidence comes forward. The advantage is that we can integrate a wide range of knowledge and therefore provide practitioners in the field with a range of options which enable them to function more effectively as rehabilitation professionals. The amount of data now available is considerable, and in many cases there are contradictory findings and different viewpoints. It seems necessary to develop some type of model so that practitioners do not have to remember vast amounts of technical knowledge but can generalize the knowledge in a logical fashion from a model which they are able to understand. In other words, models bring about comprehension, and comprehension brings about a wider band of information that can be applied within the field.

Perhaps equally important, the development of a model provides an opportunity to extrapolate in ways which are important at this time. Firstly, rehabilitation of mentally handicapped persons has developed in an isolated fashion. Its development has been insulated from other fields of rehabilitation, whether this be the field of mental health, issues associated with elderly persons, or those associated with accident victims resulting from traumas of one type or another. Secondly, results from rehabilitation have also not been extrapolated to processes in a typical environment involving typical individuals. The principles enunciated here would seem to have general application to the processes of learning of children and adults in our community. In other words, it is argued that although levels of functioning may differ between individuals, the principles of learning and development are the same. Not only is it argued that the principles can be applied within all disability groups, but these principles of development have been, for many practitioners, the guidelines for service delivery (e.g. vocational assessment and training programmes). This is in contrast to a deficiency model in which the implications for programming are built on the assumption that certain aspects of learning will never be possible, and thus adaptation would be necessary to function at a lower level of ability. It is from these principles that we can develop new ideas. This of course is the third way in which extrapolation from any model is important. It immediately suggests new ways in which experimental processes might be developed, as well as new practical techniques for dealing with individuals who are handicapped.

Of course, we should recognize that what is being described is not just about a rehabilitation process, but also refers to a basic description of how our society plans, learns and modifies its own structures and systems. Therefore the proposals we are putting forward are of a dynamic nature, and if applied broadly have relevance within the context of human society.

CHAPTER TWO

Psychological development and structure in rehabilitation

Introduction

Developmental psychology has provided, both clinically and experimentally, an overall view of the sequence of behavioural development that has practical relevance to the child or adult who, due to accident, stress or other damage, has regressed to an earlier level of performance. In such cases it has become acceptable to apply knowledge about child development in the design and application of programmes in the rehabilitation field. When the practitioner understands and systematically applies such knowledge to delivery of individualized and structured intervention, more effective changes in performance can occur. The structure consists of a sequence of interventions which are built from the results of baseline assessment and are the result of an understanding of biological, including environmental, and psychological processes. In other words, rehabilitation from an educational perspective represents, to a very large degree, a response to natural behavioural phenomena which are unacceptable given the individual's age. The process of rehabilitation therefore involves the enhancement of those structures which accelerate normal development.

Behavioural modalities and evolutionary development

Learning takes place through a variety of sensory modalities which, over the course of time, have evolved from basic and very simple sensory cells within primitive organisms. The presence of touch-sensitive and light-sensitive cells occurs in many simple organisms. From an evolutionary perspective tactile sensitivity was a precursor to light sensitivity, and light sensitivity preceded the development of auditory sense cells. Over the course of evolution specific cells have differentiated into organs which are particularly organized to deal with specific types and ranges of environmental stimulation. From the point of view of the model presented here, tactile and kinaesthetic stimulation, visual stimulation and auditory stimulation are the most relevant.

In the evolutionary sequence there is, both within a modality such as sight or sound, but also between modalities, increasing complexity as this development takes

rimates particular specialization of the visual modality for the
ment, light colour and depth perception occurs. Auditory percep-
d to a level where very detailed stimulation can be analysed to
organisms to differentiate between slight variations in sound

... volutionary point of view, modalities have developed in a specific sequence, it seems likely that a related hierarchy of development will be found within a species. Although it is too simplistic to suggest ontogeny repeats phylogeny, it is suggested that structures which come to have evolutionary valency, and are therefore necessary in the development of more advanced functions, are retained in rudimentary form during the development of a specific organism (Curtis, 1975). At a behavioural level this sequence appears to play an important role in rehabilitation programming.

The point of these introductory remarks is to indicate that evolution is a structured process. One stage follows from another stage, and the initial building block in a simpler organism which is necessary for a subsequent stage in a more advanced organism often remains, even if in rudimentary form, within the latter's developmental process. Because physical and anatomical structure follow a particular pattern, it is likely that behavioural development will correlate with this pattern in terms of sequence. Within an organism, ontogeny appears as an important process in which developmental sequences appear to be laid down with detailed relationships and interaction between behaviour and organic and environmental structure. It must be recognized that the plan is, as Lorenz (1981) suggests, a blueprint. The structures have certain basic form, but there is a degree of plasticity in behaviour which is influenced by maturation and by learning. In rehabilitation, therefore, structure in terms of the order and complexity of stimulation that is provided is likely to be critically important in the development of an effective programme.

In other words, the structure of the human organism is such that stimuli to be received and interpreted must be in a certain form, and that form must come within a specific sequence if it is to be understood, interpreted and used by the individual. The importance of this is frequently missed within the rehabilitation field at a behavioural level.

There comes a point in the individual's development where deterioration begins to occur; first slowly, and finally at a fairly fast rate. Thus beyond a certain age physical structure begins to break down. New learning becomes more difficult and more recently learnt material is readily forgotten. The process can be likened to the action of water on limestone with development of fissures, the dissolution of parts of the structure and, eventually, fall-down of the complex. The processes of regression and the forces causing development and decline in ability are schematically represented in Figure 1. The implication is that while, during the early years, rehabilitation involves building new structures, in later years the process of rehabilitation involves replacing structures that have been lost. In one sense this is artificial in that both processes go on throughout the life cycle, but the latter increasingly dominates with increasing age. It is argued that the behavioural processes involved in rehabilitation at any age are basically the same, even though the implications for the individual may be very different. The effect of ageing processes, accelerated by accident, may, for example, cause a decline of self-image to a very great degree. Failure in a child with Down's syndrome may also result in a decline in self-image.

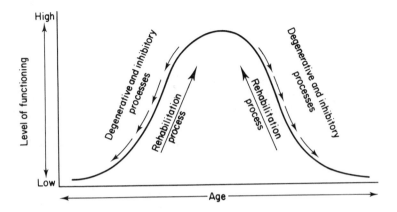

Figure 1. Schematic representation of rehabilitation and degenerative forces in relation to age.

Visual perception and rehabilitation

The structured nature of development is seen clearly within the psychology of visual perception. The phenomenon of visual constancy has been recognized and examined in experimental psychology for a long while. A child gradually develops a perceptual framework based on new and past stimuli from different modalities (Wolman, 1973).

The work of Hebb (1949) indicates the importance of the development of visual schemata in persons blind since birth, but who regain their sight in adulthood through surgical intervention. The research quoted by Hebb involved newly sighted subjects attempting to recognize such objects as circles, squares and triangles through visual presentation. Initially individuals found this impossible, and only with elaborate practice, by noting angles and sides and employing gross eye movements (e.g. focusing on each corner), could they eventually come to recognize a particular shape at a glance. This work not only underlines the slow and gradual development of visual−perceptual structures, but lends some credence to Hebb's subsequent suggestions on learning, cognition and the formation of hierarchical structures. Thus continued stimulation appears to result in a process we call learning, which has neurochemical and structural counterparts within the nervous system. Presumably such stimulation results in more regular and effective performance, and in adaptation to the environment. Thus learning becomes more and more precise, with the individual adapting increasingly to the situation in which he is functioning.

It can be argued that on the behavioural side there are psychological responses which can be arranged in a continuum from random and gross behaviour to specific and precise behaviour. On the neurological side there appear remote or random connections between neurons which, as learning takes place, change to close and specific connections which are associated with more precise and permanent behaviour.

Role of structure

From a behavioural perspective it is important, in the first instance, for the young child to develop some form of structure which acts as a reference for new infor-mation. It is also recognized that if tentative, internal structure breaks down through removal to an unfamiliar or new environment the child shows some breakdown in visual structuring. On return to the original environment a very young child shows disturbed behaviour such as the phenomenon of global gazing (Schaeffer, 1963). The same behaviour has been observed by Brown (1965) in studies of older but retarded youngsters. In these instances the individual moved to a new environment becomes very quiet, the range of spontaneous verbal statements diminishes and there are changes in visuo-motor behaviour. The latter includes an increase in stereotyped movements, a reduction in accurate item manipulation and placement, and may also include global gazing or searching. It is as if the child is searching for stability. Hutt, Hutt and Ounstead (1965) describe the behaviour of young normal and disabled children in unfamiliar environments, specifically in relation to play. Again stereotyped movements, sometimes tentative investigation of the environment and tactile response to items within the room, occur. Toys may be ignored and the child is unlikely to concentrate upon them. Yet a familiar adult standing by the toys is sufficient to encourage play for a longer period of time. Familiar physical and social structures seem important to very young children, and without them behav-iour emission rate is reduced and attention to specific items becomes short-term. It is suggested that in normal children the phenomena described relate to age, because young age is associated with new learning which involves reduced attention span. Since the same phenomenon can be seen with older disabled children it would appear that the important factor is the degree of new learning which is involved rather than chronological age *per se*.

But there are other examples suggesting that structure is mediated by adults in the child's environment, and seems critical for learning. Holding a child's hand and preventing his responses while encouraging thinking improves accuracy of response (Haywood, 1985). Luria (1961) noted the shift from the child being controlled by an adult's speech to the child being controlled by his own speech. This developmen-tal sequence is the rationale for self-instructional training procedures which require the child first to imitate the adult's guiding verbalization and then supply his own (Meichenbaum and Goodman, 1971).

There is other evidence which supports a structured process being developed within the learning system. Douglas and Blomfield (1949) have shown that young children, under 5 years of age, who remain in a familiar family environment, show less breakdown than children who change environment as a result of, for example, mother entering hospital. It would appear that as early as 1949 there was some recognition that stability of physical environment was of immense importance to a young child, and that disruption of behaviour would occur if major changes occurred to this environment. This aspect of learning is taken up in later chapters, but at this point it is important to stress the likely importance of permanent or semi-permanent external structures in the development of the young child's learning.

All of these studies suggest that predictable and physically familiar structures are extremely important in facilitating a young child's or a disabled child's learning and adaptive processes. The fact that at a later age such familiarity and physical stimulation are normally less necessary suggests that whatever processes or characteristics are in the external environment, they are no longer so necessary as learning progresses.

One model to account for this change is that external processes have been replicated in some form within the central nervous system and the individual can now depend on these, albeit unconsciously, as reference points in order to gauge the external environment. Although this is not the same as the phenomenon of visual constancy, it nevertheless has something in common with it; namely, when learning has not been internalized, as the external field loses its reference points, an individual starts increasing the magnitude of error in making assessments and eventually behaviour breaks down. The more experienced the individual (i.e. the more learning that has taken place), the less the number of cues that are necessary in the environment in order to perform accurately or retain stable behaviour.

There are at least two types of stimuli loss in the field of disability: (1) where the environment may lose its range and magnitude of stimulation (e.g. when institutionalization occurs), and (2) when the individual's sensory and internal nervous systems break down so that the individual is less capable of receiving such stimulation. The two phenomena often go together, each acting on the other resulting in further and major deterioration (see later).

It would appear under these circumstances that there are likely to be critical thresholds where an individual becomes confused and disabled, firstly in terms of learning, since new stimuli are involved, and then in terms of routine behaviour which becomes disrupted. It is also more likely that the more established the learning, and therefore the fewer external cues that are required to maintain its operation, the less likely it is to be disrupted by adverse external or internal events. By the same token one would assume that if the learning system is well embedded in the behavioural repertoire due to a high level of repetition, there will have to be a large amount of loss or damage to internal nervous tissue before such well-established learning is disrupted.

Although the examples given are from the field of visual information, it is suggested that they are equally relevant to the field of tactile and auditory stimulation, and that continuing performance and maintenance is likely to be related to the period when the learning took place. The earlier in life a process is learned, the more likely it is to be maintained, although there are exceptions. Tactile learning is likely to be better established than visual, and visual rather better than auditory.

In simplistic terms, first learned material will be retained and employed after later learned material has been disrupted.

Early learning—the route to structure

In his early work on the organization of human behaviour Hebb (1949) posited two types of learning—one referred to as early learning, the other as later learning. Early learning was defined as a process which normally takes place in the early years of life and occurs less often in later years where later learning or transfer phenomena tend to occur. Early learning is original learning. It requires a large number of stimuli—response connections before it is properly attained and is subject to over-generalization. Later learning, because it is essentially made up of previously learned material, which is reorganized for new operations, does not take long, and is fast and effective learning.

There are a number of questions related to these two processes in normal human learning; one being whether early learning or original learning can take place in older persons. Increasingly, in an era where we see the development of continuing education for the senior citizen, it is supposed that original learning can be generated over much of life, although questions about the amount of transfer involved in this process arise.

It is important to know whether such learning can take place in the disabled adult. The disabled adult is often at a stage where early learning is required—either because the person has suffered since birth from genetic or environmental conditions, resulting in damage to the nervous system, so that the individual has never attained sufficient early learned skills, or because the individual, having received damage at a later stage, has lost a wide range of early learned skills. Since later learning involves the selection of appropriate blocks of learned material from previous experience, the ability to do this selection appropriately is of some consequence. Since learning becomes more refined and sophisticated with experience, it is likely that the transfer phenomenon can be a more precise process with increasing age. Indeed casual observation suggests that the wider the range of specific learning in a particular area (e.g. use of transit skills), the more effective will be the transfer or generalization effects. The nature of disability is such that specific learning is slower and disability itself is associated with environmental restrictions. Both factors reduce the likelihood of positive transfer effects.

These factors are often not taken into account in rehabilitation programmes. For example, when teaching a particular social skill it is necessary to identify the learning structures so that the specific components are learned. This leads to transfer training carried out in various environmental contexts. This means that in rehabilitation programmes considerable analysis of components in specific skills is required, bearing in mind the environmental situations in which the skills will be employed. For example to teach someone to respond to a greeting appropriately needs: (a) teaching of a verbal component, (b) a body position component, (c) facial responsiveness which is consistent with the verbal response, (d) environmental context, (e) time of the interaction, (f) familiarity with the person, and so on. It involves teaching a wide range of specific responses which can be combined in different ways, depending on the situation, thus requiring the trainer to provide a wide diversity of environmental structures for effective use.

Unfortunately practitioners often teach the verbal response appropriate to a greeting in a training centre or school where the environment is restricted. Thus a variety of components are ignored, leaving the student with a very rigid, artificial and non-transferable piece of behaviour.

Early learning and disability

If the individual is handicapped from birth the early learning phenomenon may need to take place at other stages of life. Further, the slower the learning the greater the likelihood of greater magnitude of observed variability over time between individuals. This is consistent with the data of variability provided by Gunzburg (1968) (see Figure 12).

A period of early learning not only involves the emission of gross behavioural responses. Over-generalization begins to occur so that individuals react to more than the required, specific stimuli and apply their learning in inappropriate situations (Sluckin, 1964). For example, an ability to give the name of a bearded adult may first be demonstrated by the application of that name to all men with beards before it is applied solely to the appropriate man with a beard. Only with further training will the individual cease to over-generalize and apply responses in the specific and appropriate instances. This is an important concept, for it shows that individuals who begin to over-generalize are learning. It can also be shown that the phenomenon of over-generalization is one that becomes inhibited as effective learning proceeds.

Paradoxically, the opposite problem to over-generalization is often encountered in the rehabilitation process; namely, once a task has been learned, there is a lack of appropriate generalization or transfer of responses to other relevant situations. The problem is that many rehabilitation personnel attempt to teach specific skills only. This limits the generalization process which has an important role in community living. Indeed many teachers and trainers complain that once a task is learned the individual fails to produce the necessary behaviour in different but appropriate situations. It seems that much vocational training and occupational therapy is associated with the teaching of specific tasks. Yet Gold (1973), Clarke and Clarke (1974), and many others have indicated the importance of training for transfer. But the nature of much rehabilitation training is to teach people how not to transfer. Thus in situations like specific skill training, where we use formal means to inhibit over-generalization, it is highly unlikely that clients will be able to employ transfer or generalization when it is relevant.

Gold argues that most rehabilitation programmes only expose people to transfer situations. That is, it is assumed that once specific skills have been learned the individual will transfer the skill effectively in a new environment or slightly modified task situation. However, if generalization or transfer processes become inhibited in early learning, it is essential that a planned and structured approach be initiated by the trainer to promote transfer of skills.

Clarke and Blakemore (1961) and Clarke and Cookson (1962) carried out a series of experiments on transfer and noted that many handicapped children and adults, although moderately mentally retarded, showed effective transfer on a variety of learning tasks. The tasks used in their experiments were essentially of a spatial perceptual nature. As noted above, teachers have, for example, claimed that transfer is poor amongst mentally handicapped children. But there may be a critical difference between experimental transfer and the classroom situation. It so happens that in the Clarke and Cookson and the Clarke and Blakemore experiments, the authors employed highly structured learning sequences in order to have rigid experimental control. Accidentally, and perhaps incidentally, an excellent structured transfer training situation was also provided. The experimenters defined the type of room in which the experiments were to take place, the nature of the specific materials and verbal instructions were also carefully arranged. In rehabilitation situations this structured approach to transfer rarely occurs.

Time, place and stimulation

In order for development to proceed effectively the right stimuli have to be present at the right time. In a normal environment these stimuli tend to be readily available, and such stimuli are highlighted by the presence of relevant others who highlight the stimuli, or increase their availability for the child at each stage of development. As Skinner (1957) has noted, at particular stages parents and teachers intensify specific learning processes. They may do this by repeatedly drawing attention to specific aspects of an environment (e.g. pointing to and naming a dog) or by enriching the environment with specific stimuli (e.g. particular toys at specific stages of development). It can also be done by particular movements from the adult in relation to the learning material. For example, Hutt, Hutt and Ounstead demonstrated that in unfamiliar environments a familiar adult standing by toys promoted play with those toys.

By and large such behaviour appears to be based on accumulated wisdom in a society through, for example, modelling teaching behaviour, such as parents applying knowledge from their own past experience with their own parents. But as society becomes more sophisticated and aware of learning processes it devises more specific experiences for children at particular ages. For example McConkey and Jeffree (1981) advise on selection of toys for children of specific ages and abilities. Unfortunately society at times forgets or loses the accumulated wisdom. For example, many rhymes that have been employed over a long period are not known to many parents in the current generation. Bryant and Bradley (1985) point to the important association between learning disabilities in reading and the absence of rhyme. It appears that rhyme plays an important role in the structured development of reading and allied skills. It also represents a developmental experience which seems to be a necessary pre-reading skill.

In general terms, specialized or enriched stimulation is based on an age expectancy model—on average neither too early nor too late—although between generations some flexibility is apparent. For example, young adults are currently provided with car driving instruction during the teens, but 40 years ago the average for instruction was probably around 30 years of age. There are also age variations between countries and cultures. This latter variation suggests that a knowledge of culture-based stimuli should be taken into account in interpreting the nature of disabilities. This is particularly true where a country has a mixed and changing cultural heritage. For example the immigration of families from Africa and the West Indies to Western countries resulted in many of their children being sent to special schools for mentally handicapped children; a phenomenon which would be expected to slow down social integration processes.

It is recognized that learning is a lifelong process, and with advances in technology it is accepted that a range of new skills will need to be taught within a society (e.g. computer literacy). Yet our society has still not accepted that this is also necessary within the rehabilitation field. Indeed in rehabilitation the situation is much worse since most agencies, particularly for adults, are technologically 'behind the times'. For example, out-of-date printing presses are employed in some vocational shops which use vastly different skills from those needed in the modern print industry. Little is done to overcome such skill differences in the vocational rehabilitation model in preparing people for employment. This lack of appropriate stimulation for skill developments results in employment failure which is erroneously perceived as a function of disability.

Another aspect of age variation is seen in relation to decline or lack of attainment in certain developmental skills. For example inability to remember where one lives, dressing inappropriately for weather conditions, drooling and inability to feed oneself, are seen as unacceptable behaviour in adults and children of a certain age. It becomes a question of whether the necessary training stimuli are available to overcome such problems during the rehabilitation process. This requires an examination of individual needs, and is a matter which reflects on the philosophy of programming and the skills of staff. If no appropriate opportunities exist within the programme, the disability may simply be one of programme limitation. In many situations such behaviours are accepted as signs of inappropriate responsiveness, but mechanisms are not brought into play to deal with the situation. The responsibility therefore lies with the programme design and development, not with the individual who shows the problem.

Structure and behavioural components—concluding comments

The discussion has indicated that several hierarchical or structured systems occur in the learning, and therefore in the rehabilitation process. One illustrates development through tactile, visual to auditory modalities while a second defines the sequence of development within a modality. It is suggested that the most recently developed modality will be the most easily damaged, and the most advanced and complex operations within a modality are those most easily damaged or affected by stress events. It might be reasonable to predict that auditory malfunctioning will be more common than visual, and that visual problems will be more common than tactile in cases where general CNS deterioration occurs in certain conditions of physical trauma (e.g. anoxia, teratogens), viral infection or even long-term decline in motivation. The law of 'last in first out' should apply. It might be expected that linguistic components would be more easily disrupted than visual components unless very specific brain injury or sensory damage is involved. Within the auditory modality refined aspects of language would be expected to deteriorate before more gross auditory phenomena.

The third system, which is closely related, represents the nature of environmental structure in the development of new learning and the gradual internalization of knowledge, which means that the individual comes to impose structure on his or her environment. This is an important principle for rehabilitation, but the process is not complete unless effective transfer training can be accomplished. It is noted that normal environments supply a range of stimuli which society (frequently parents or teachers) highlight as children approach new developmental stages. Because disability implies that people may show a breakdown in typical 'readiness times' the rehabilitation practitioner must structure the environmental stimuli so they are appropriate for a disabled individual functioning at a specific level within a particular programme area.

It seems likely that the first signs of breakdown or stress will be observed in new learning, because new learning will normally represent the most advanced stage of a person's activity. But the later stages of learning are generally built on previously learned materials, thus material which is learned later is generally more complex. Thus a further continuum in the developmental sphere is represented by the simple to complex nature of the learning continuum.

Many of the behaviours which are regarded as a disability are not abnormal in themselves. The process may occur in all humans but is regarded as unacceptable when it is not age-appropriate. For example, everyone shows slips of the tongue, especially when fatigued or under stress. Generally such behaviour is transitory and the individual tends to recognize the error. When this behaviour is emitted by a disabled person it is seen as an abnormal phenomenon. It is often seen as a sign of low intelligence. Such behaviour frequently occurs in accident victims, who have suffered neurological damage, and also occurs in elderly persons who are suffering neural system deterioration. Although frequency of the behaviour is relevant to whether or not the characteristic is regarded as abnormal, it must be recognized that occurrence of the behaviour is not simply an abnormal process, for it occurs in all people at some time. It is a normal process in the environment-person exchange. Yet it is statistically more common and persistent in those who have disabilities. The point is to comprehend why it occurs and when it occurs, in order to devise processes to correct or reduce the phenomenon. It would seem that most normal individuals can correct the behaviour through immediate feedback. Where it has reached abnormal statistical frequency the use of a variety of meta-cognitive processes, and the application of specific learning principles, should assist in correcting the problem. It is a combination of these principles and other structures which form one part of programme design in the rehabilitation process.

CHAPTER THREE

The development of rehabilitation programme continua

Introduction

The case for developing stuctured programmes seems to be overwhelming. For more than two decades various programmes and procedures have been developed, many of which claim to be effective with handicapped children (Bronfenbrenner, 1975; Bricker, Seibert and Casuso, 1980) and adults (Halpern, 1973; Clarke and Clarke, 1974; Hughson, Berrien and Brown, 1978; Brown and Hughson, 1980; Ward *et al.*, 1981; Sykes and Smith, 1984). Although many handicapped persons now remain in the community, and a large number obtain employment, very little of the programme development has been put into a comprehensive model of rehabilitation. In this chapter two major themes are developed:

1. An examination of aspects of lifestyle and a formulation of the constituent components of rehabilitation into a series of programme areas or continua.
2. A discussion of the internal structures involved in each programme area with a description of the developmental sequence involved.

The concept of programme continua

The model of rehabilitation being proposed involves a number of primary features. First there is a recognition that mental handicap, mental illness and physical disability are the result of a variety of interacting primary and secondary negative impacts. But each individual is not only subjected to negative situations or events, for primary and secondary positive impacts also occur. It is argued that, in order to understand the rehabilitation process and to apply an effective model of rehabilitation to each individual, these positive and negative impacts must be recognized and detailed at the programme-building stage for each individual. They represent in one sense the quality that recognizes that each individual is unique, and determine for that individual a specialized and independent programme.

A second requirement relates not so much to the individual *per se*, but to the nature of rehabilitation programming, for there appears to be a structured hierarchy which can be viewed in the framework of several continua (see Figure 2).

Rehabilitation procedures provide the basic rules upon which any continuous rehabilitation programme can be built, but these have to be applied at different levels. These levels are the steps within the continua.

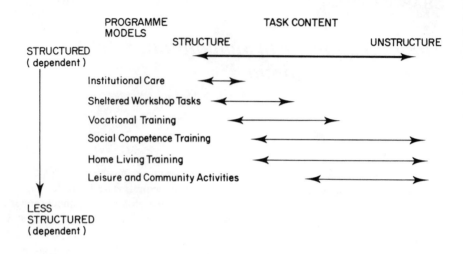

Figure 2. The dimension of structure in relation to programme models and task content.

There also appear to be concrete and abstract developmental processes, and in normal development these are recognized by a variety of research workers (e.g. Piaget, 1952a; Piaget and Inhelder, 1956; Kagan and Moss, 1962). This sequence of developmental steps can be arranged into a longitudinal plan and divided into areas of functioning (e.g. vocational, social). The process relates to how an individual's sequence of learning interfaces within different areas of environmental stimulation and represents the areas in which individuals function. Thus the area continua, as they may be called, have their roots in human developmental sequences; indeed the two, i.e. human development and programme continua, must parallel one another.

In rehabilitation a knowledge of these continua is critical, and for the most part, in rehabilitation, they heighten but follow the natural developmental sequences of growing youngsters. At times they deviate from this path because of the specific nature of particular types of handicapping conditions. Yet they remain a plausible guide to interpreting behavioural functioning. Not only are these continua arranged from concrete to abstract levels of development, but they also represent a process of external to internalized behaviour. Of course none of the continua are discrete, but represent approximate areas of functioning which interrelate one with the other.

Historical development of training continua institutions

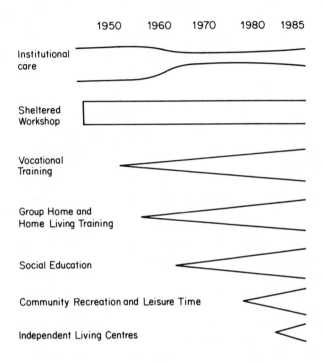

Figure 3. Changing nature of rehabilitation.

In order to understand the origins of these continua (see Figure 3) it is necessary to look at the development of rehabilitation services. A brief review of the history of rehabilitation services over the past 100 years suggests that until about 1950, although there were some differences between communities, institutional care was the rule of the day, with large hospitals built in remote rural areas. The institutions were often designated for individuals suffering from particular types of disorder as recognized particularly within the medical community at the time, such as cerebral palsy, epilepsy and the various levels of mental deficiency. The reasons for such care were complex and related to:

1. the provision of care and living facilities for handicapped children and adults, and
2. the need to protect society.

During the second half of the twentieth century the notion that many institutionalized individuals were not dissimilar from others in the community became accepted by the public. In some cases persons were sent to hospitals through errors of medical, social and/or legal decision. For example, an individual having committed a minor crime, living within a poor family structure with economic poverty, would frequently be given a verbal test of intelligence. The results of such tests would often be well below average because of the low level of verbal stimulation within which the individual lived. Courts would, on this basis, decide the individual was mentally deficient and therefore, rather than 'punishing the crime', would determine that a mental deficiency hospital represented an appropriate placement for the individual. This form of placement and incarceration was questioned during the 1950s.

Concerns over these issues arose amongst the various civil liberty groups, but this period also saw the rise in Scandinavia of the normalization movement which advocated access to normal lifestyles for handicapped persons (Nirje, 1970). The normalization movement, which has been largely accepted from a conceptual and philosophical point of view, is attuned to the social attitudes of human rights. Yet society, and particularly the educational, health and welfare services have not effectively built the basic rehabilitation structures that are necessary for making such a philosophy a success. In some instances the technology exists, but has not been comprehensively or consistently applied. Thus the need for an effective model of rehabilitation. The concept of normalization, which included helping handicapped persons forward in a stepwise process along the road to normal functioning, was elaborated by Wolfensberger and Glenn (1975), who argued that the philosophy applied to a wide range of persons who were deviant in terms of the 'normal' community. Both these concepts, i.e. a stepwise approach to progress towards normality and the application of the normalization principle to all disabled groups, are critical to the arguments put forward in this book. Indeed, the recognition by Wolfensberger that the philosophical principles of normalization within the rehabilitation field have generic application represented one of the first attempts to promote an integrated approach to disability. That the commonality of problems is becoming accepted is seen in an article in *Social Work Today*, advocating the application of group home procedures in the field of mental handicap to allied procedures in the area of mental health (Brendon, 1984).

As a result of the movement described above, the past three decades have seen a marked decrease in institutionalization, not only in terms of admission to institutions, but also in the reintegration of people from institutions into the normal society. In many communities such development has proceeded rapidly, supported by parents' movements, and more recently by various advocacy organizations (e.g. People First). Such developments, although associated to some considerable degree with mental retardation, have also occurred in the area of mental illness, and are now being considered in the field of ageing (Cohen and Dickerson, 1983; Janicki and Wisniewski, 1985).

Despite these advances, the first signs of a trend in the opposite direction were observed during the late 1970s and early 1980s. That is not to say that deinstitutionalization has been stopped, but rather in its headlong rush we see the beginnings of resistance and some movement towards reinstitutionalization, e.g. ageing mentally handicapped persons being moved into institutional settings, setting up of small institutions for profoundly retarded persons, non-community placement of people from vocational training agencies. The reasons for this relate only in part to our knowledge about handicap, but are more critically associated with the prevailing economic and political *zeitgeist*. These items will be discussed later, but it is important to recognize that, without a clear understanding of the political and economic conditions within any environment, it is unlikely that rehabilitation will be effective (Brown, 1984b). Further, until rehabilitation develops a sound theoretical framework it will continue to be directed by the transient whims of political and social popularism, or be perceived as a set of technical practices.

One of the major reasons for the deinstitutionalization movement relates to the poor care in, and condition of, many hospitals. It is incorrect to think that people were placed in such institutions with the idea of providing inadequate care. Indeed the opposite was the case, at least in the mind of those who at the time observed the squalid and devastating condition lived in by many individuals within the urban communities of Europe and North America. Society, at different times, through various individuals, was concerned that the highest level of care be provided (Sloan and Stevens, 1976; Sarason and Doris, 1979). The community environment from which individuals frequently came was atrocious, and any improvement and respite offered by institutions, by comparison, made such places seem civilized ventures at the time they were designed. This is not to suggest institutions were places of benign care. The nature of mental illness, for example, before the advent of barbiturates, often saw the accumulation of a mass of disturbed humanity in restricting conditions under the rule of unenlightened personnel. The passage of time, coupled with social change and the fact that such settings were not clearly monitored by an unbiased society, led to their increasing unpopularity and their gradual downfall. Examples relating to enquiries into institutional practice abound, such as the case of Willowbrook (Wortis, 1981). Yet this in itself is a simplification. Forces to control abuse were set up in most areas, and an attempt was made to ensure that individuals were provided with effective care, although this did not mean returning individuals to society. Even in our literature both the benign and the bestial have been exemplified by such writers as Trollop and Dickens, and we would do well to remember the complexities and conflicting forces in these early years. However, despite efforts to control abuse in institutions for handicapped persons, such centres continue, and at times are still associated with dehumanizing practices.

Vocational training

After the Second World War occupational therapy and vocational training programmes became a feature of hospitals, and a variety of other private agencies followed these developments. Some were directed to improving skills, but many of them were make-work programmes to keep individuals active, and in some cases they were referred to as activity centres. The term 'sheltered workshop' was often used, as subcontracts from factories became part of the routine of some of these agencies. Many of them designed their own types of production relating to products such as horticultural equipment, flower boxes, tables and chairs, and very often the key jobs were taken over by staff, with some of the minor jobs, such as sanding and painting, being carried out by the clients. Gradually such experiences led some to think that work could be provided on a more meaningful basis, and that, with training, individuals could become competitively employed in the outside community. Certainly this was the feature of work developed by O'Connor and Tizard (1956) and by Clarke and Clarke (1974) in Britain. In the United States attitudinal change was more an offshoot of some of the vocational and sheltered workshops for physically disabled persons returning from the Second World War.

Work, and later meaningful work, was seen as a necessary process for helping handicapped people. It was a logical development in institutions for handicapped people. In many cases the hospitals had a ready supply of work in kitchens, laundries, and in the largely self-supporting agricultural activities. Yet in most cases, as demonstrated in *A Century of Concern* (Sloan and Stevens, 1976) describing a hundred years of the American Association on Mental Deficiency, it was not considered that individuals would grow and develop to the point where they could take a remunerative place in the community. The phenomenon of vocational occupation and, prior to that, sheltered workshops or work programmes, was that they were primarily time-fillers and secondly vocational training settings.

It was within this context during the 1950s and 1960s that a variety of programmes were developed which applied principles of learning, involving more effective training techniques. The early programmes carried out in Britain, and later by Gold (1973) in the United States, Brown and Hughson (1980) and Marlett and Hughson (1977) in Canada, and Parmenter (1983) in Australia, showed how the particular processes could be applied effectively to raise performance levels of clients. In many instances they were a demonstration of the fact that handicapped persons, even severely handicapped persons, could learn tasks effectively even though they had been institutionalized for many years. Learning, for example, could be accelerated by reward and presentation of a task in small units and in brief time periods. Yet many of these individuals who had been trained did not make their way into the outside community. Some were essentially subjects in vocational experiments who demonstrated, with the help of their experimenters, that they were capable of learning. These same programme personnel, supported by the concerns of distressed parents, began to see a separation between sheltered and occupational workshops and vocational training programmes. A training continuum was beginning to take shape. Exposure to work was being replaced by a process of training which was represented by a series of developmental steps accelerated by the application of learning principles.

Although such practice is now fairly commonplace, there were (and still are) a large number of agencies that did not apply these steps or principles or, even if they knew of them, did not apply them in a consistent manner. Thus divergence amongst the infant rehabilitation programmes began to occur. A gap between research and practice was taking place. A difference between agency philosophy and procedure was occurring but had not been formally noted. The process of aligning philosophy, management and rehabilitation practice would develop at a much later stage (Brown, 1986a).

Two features of vocational work are readily apparent. First, Western society was preoccupied with a work ethic. To have work was said to give man dignity, and individuals who were handicapped could show themselves to be more like others, and thus raise their status, as they carried out work regardless of how menial or below their potential this might be. Even today much work carried out in vocational agencies and sheltered workshops is negatively value-laden and denies the notion of social role valorization advocated by Wolfensberger (1983). For example, in a recent vocational task evaluation, making coffins was seen as more profitable and long-lasting than manufacturing computer components, and therefore seen as a more desirable contract from the perspective of the vocational agency. The opposite conclusion would be arrived at when considering client self-image and societal perception.

Second, vocational training, in terms of work skills, must be regarded basically as a concrete operation. It involves routine and structure. It requires visual demonstration and tangible reinforcement. It generally takes place in one setting. More sophisticated employment options are becoming available to disabled persons, but much of the introduction to work takes the forms outlined above. In passing it should be noted that the development of concrete routines for vocational training were important skills both for the clients and the vocational staff. It is critical to understand this stage of development in order to progress to more advanced programme options. Such initial development is relatively concrete in terms of our thought processes, and for a while it was seen as an adequate method of dealing with the lives of people who were either institutionalized or permanently cared for by their relatives.

Work was often routine—that is, manual operations—and tools were put in front of an individual who had to carry out very specific procedures on a repetitive basis. There was little room for individual decision-making. There was close monitoring, and close control of the behaviours that were required. The experience thus conformed to a visual, concrete operational type of procedure. It seemed to be effective for a very large number of mentally handicapped persons. Yet over the years, as policy planners continued with the practice of segregated workshops, the problems of housing and training disabled persons continued. All existing spaces were utilized so that large numbers of people remained in 'holding tanks' or underwent the process of 'getting ready to move out', but never really moved. Thus a dilemma was created in that there were few programme spaces available for those disabled children becoming adults and insufficient funds to duplicate programmes. Today these restrictions have pushed some professionals to consider more creative options.

These points are not made with any sense of criticism, but merely to illustrate that the developmental patterns in rehabilitation commenced with containment and gradually advanced to a concrete, but limited, form of intervention. Some advances occurred and led to a more abstract concept of service. This was limited in scope in that only one aspect of lifestyle was dealt with, and it was limited in numbers to whom it could apply; it was largely disability-specific and was not future-oriented. This latter point refers to the fact that the developers of vocational programmes paid little attention in practice to what happened to individuals over the long term. A study by McKerracher (1984) indicates that outcome was for many individuals strictly limited. The evidence on the community effectiveness of vocational programming when used as a single process is still largely absent (Jackson, 1984). Yet the process did allow many individuals to enter the normal community for the first time, and foreshadowed the development of more sophisticated programmes. Even so, many jurisdictions did not develop vocational programmes, and even today there are many areas where institutional care, in one form or another, is the mainstay of the rehabilitation service system.

Vocational programming started a movement from what may be described as temporally 'near' to temporally 'distant' forms of intervention. That is, training was initially related to concrete and present situations, whereas more advanced training should prepare people for contingencies which may occur some time after training. However, this is not to suggest that historically earlier forms of intervention should be left behind or ignored, for concrete operations form a basic step in the rehabilitation process. It may, however, be that the method of application, and particularly the time of application, of such concrete operations should change quite dramatically. The processes that are outlined above tended to work primarily because they fitted into the baseline performances of many of the individuals who were in need. There does not yet seem to be any accurately predictable upper limit to the type of vocational skill that can be taught to disabled individuals, providing that we have adequate time to do so, and staff are prepared to put forward detailed task analyses along with learning strategies for teaching these tasks. The limitations lie with the programme or learning environment and the staff, *not* with the disabled person.

Within the area of physical handicap the sheltered workshops were already well established, and it is not a distant step from this to look at the area of vocational training. The point is that vocational training is largely a concrete skill. For example individuals are provided with particular materials and are required to assemble them according to a specific pattern. During the Second World War years many mentally handicapped people were employed to repair roads and carry out other activities. There was already some recognition that at least a few of these individuals were capable of organized work provided, as Tredgold (1949) indicated, they were under supervision.

The following represent some of the features that apply to a concrete operational task in the vocational area:

1. The task can be seen and touched, therefore it can be manipulated.
2. The materials are normally put together for use in a specific sequence.
3. The task is of limited duration.
4. The process is regularly repeated, often under the pressure to produce at speed.
5. There are specific tools and operational procedures which have to be followed.
6. The work is of a routine nature
7. The work is normally done in one place, which is specially designed for the purpose and does not require the individual to move around.
8. If machinery is involved it is of a standard type which has, as a rule, appropriate protective guards.

9. The work flow is organized and presented to worker (client) rather than regulated by the worker.
10. Few decisions are required by the worker regarding quality control or accuracy.

Such work can be easily learned because there are specific steps and because it is repetitive. A simple demonstration will in many cases be sufficient to show individuals how to do it. Speed can be easily increased by the use of various rewards. The application of psychological procedures such as task breakdown and the use of reward systems is clearly examined in a series of experiments carried out by Clarke and Hermelin (1955). More recently it has been recognized that a large number of multiple and severely handicapped individuals can accurately carry out much more complex tasks if appropriate task (i.e. content) analyses, and process task analyses, which include the application of individual teaching strategies, are carried out. The work of Gold (1973) and Whelan and Speake (1979) provide examples of this. In Gold's studies deaf, blind persons who were severely mentally handicapped carried out various assembly tasks.

Rehabilitation in the vocational system has started from very concrete tasks of an easy kind to more complex tasks, which require greater analysis, but also greater knowledge on the part of the client and the teacher. We therefore have a continuum which is shown within Figure 3. The complex assembly tasks that Gold has advocated are represented at the wider end of the continuum. They suggest that not only are tasks for mentally handicapped persons more complicated than they used to be when vocational rehabilitation started, but a wider range of handicapped persons carry them out. Within the vocational training continuum itself there are a number of complex variables. These relate to the task itself, including sequencing of its components, the ability of the trainer to carry out task analysis and apply teaching strategies, the range of handicapped persons that can be served and the supports available in the environment.

Social education training

As vocational programmes multiplied, mentally handicapped people began to be placed in employment. This started during the 1950s, but work failure often occurred. This happened for a variety of reasons. Although some individuals lacked vocational skills for particular employment, and inappropriate job placements were made, other reasons were predominant. As early as 1961 Earl, and later, Gunzburg (1960, 1968), recognized the importance of social rehabilitation, and the latter recognized the importance of social educational skills in the preparation of handicapped young adults for vocational placements. In data on vocational performance, failures often appeared to occur in social skill areas (Esgrow, 1978), rather than in areas of actual work performance (Brown, Bayer and MacFarlane, 1985). This recognition has led to a plethora of social educational programmes, and in North America to a revision of special education curricula to include this aspect of skill training.

Social educational, social living skills, aids to daily living (ADL), or life skills need to be recognized and taught. At first rehabilitation personnel concentrated on academic education which was perceived as socially and vocationally relevant. In other words the interpretation was conceptually concrete. For example, reading and simple mathematics skills were perceived as important, but this gave way to the more practical social sight vocabularies (i.e. recognizing what to do when certain words or symbols are presented, e.g. Danger, Stop). Simple budgeting skills and making change were eventually regarded as appropriate substitutes to mathematics education. Indeed it was believed that teaching such skills would meet clients' basic needs. It is of interest that the more formal educational characteristics or activities proved difficult to learn compared with the social educational skills. The characteristics appear to relate to comments by McKerracher *et al.* (1980) regarding the notion that achievement in educational skills appears to be positively correlated with intelligence measures. Further, social skills have more immediate practical value and appear meaningful to the client, whereas a formal educational curriculum is more remote, long-term and thus, abstract.

The social educational continuum is also conceived as starting from basic concrete skills, such as word recognition, through expansion of language and concepts of number, to more formal educational skills in reading and writing, beginning with practical abilities such as signing one's name. The application of these skills in a variety of community areas is also viewed as part of the continuum. The interpersonal nature of these skills as they become developed must also be included within the continuum because it is important not only to have such skills, but to be able to apply them in a variety of community-relevant situations. It is necessary to learn and over-learn certain basic skills before they can be applied and used efficiently in the community in a varied and spontaneous manner. For example a knowledge of number and coin recognition precedes budgeting and shopping procedures, but as the latter begin to develop, self-awareness and self-assertive skills are required to deal with varied and changing situations which involve estimation and challenges made by other community individuals. Thus we begin to see the importance of building into the process skills of variability and generalization. The continuum starts with specific skill training and terminates with generalizable application.

Such a continuum must involve self-assertiveness training, including the growth of social maturity to confront and effectively deal with challenging situations in the environment. This leads quite naturally into the area of sexuality training. In one sense this introduction is artificial since it frequently is begun at an adult stage. It may be more appropriate to phase in a number of the basic concepts and skills relating to personal development at earlier stages of self-awareness and self-concept (Johnson, 1984). However, handicapped individuals with poor self-image often come to agencies at older ages, and self-image can often be boosted by first providing a number of basic and useful community skills. This is seen quite clearly with learning-disabled children who may find it difficult to read and have developed poor self-image. It is hard to bolster self-image unless positive development occurs in relation to the basic problem in front of them— in the case of learning-disabled persons, reading.

Social education covers a wide range of skills such as budgeting, time management, transportation and social sight reading, to name a few. Increased understanding of social educational need was such that by the beginning of the 1970s many programmes had developed basic social educational training. Yet many government officials of that time, who were responsible for funding such programmes, did not understand why such education had to be blended with vocational training. Concrete thinking in adults is not restricted to disabled persons! It occurs with everyone—the principles are the same, the levels different.

Home living training

It is perhaps fair to suggest that residential training other than through institutional care started somewhat earlier than social education training, but the use of the variety of group homes that are seen in the development of fairly sophisticated normalized home living environments within the community is of more recent origin. Initially, group homes were simply places where handicapped people lived. Gradually they were viewed as training environments. Therefore they represented more than a 'home' situation. Such homes are now developed across a wide range of disability groups, and residential care, utilizing home skill training, has become a regular programme for many atypical children and adults, including those with mental handicap, behavioural disturbance and antisocial and criminal behaviour (Fewster and Garfat, 1987).

Traditionally the skills have been referred to as residential but it is more appropriate to label these as home living skills. It is not just a matter of changing a name, but recognizing that rehabilitation is not concerned so much with residential care, although this may be involved, but with the development of home skills which can be applied within community settings. The aim is to promote the teachings of adaptive skills in high-quality learning environments. Such units often involve no more than five people in each setting. At the lower end of this continuum the skills involve a large component of motor and attentional abilities. Comprehension of the skills, either through tactile direction, visual modelling or auditory command, are also involved. There is a difference between these instruction forms in terms of hierarchy, and one type of instruction may be more appropriate than another at certain stages of development (see later). The continuum moves through personal routines that the client requires to maintain himself or herself in the community, but fairly quickly in the development of the continuum there is transfer from externalized behaviour and control, involving copying or interpreting commands, to an internal schedule where the individual produces behaviour through his or her own instigation. This, again, is a feature of all the continua and the development of a system of external to internal structuring is critical to rehabilitation. However, external controls are generally more apparent in the vocational continuum than in the other continua, probably accounting for the early development and relative ease of training in the vocational domain. Personal routines, such as washing and dressing, may be followed by more complex skills associated with home management. Individuals move on to semi-independence in apartment training and eventually live on their own.

In both the areas of social education and group home living, a range of skills is taught, and the skills appear to be rather more abstract than those in the vocational area. If a mentally disabled person is asked if he or she would like a lift in a car, the decision that is made is not one involving major motor movements, but a process of internalized judgement and decision-making. Further, there are a range of specific times and places when such events are likely to occur. The events themselves have consequences which may place an individual in new and unusual situations. In this sense social tasks are often of an abstract nature. Furthermore, because of the various places in which such behaviours take place, the likelihood of having a supervisor or foreman present is remote. The only means for decision-making lies with the individual concerned. Even here there is variation. For example, an individual wishes to learn how to buy clothes. It is important to begin with concrete decisions requiring minimal judgement in order to build confidence and competence which will be needed for more complex social judgements. This example is a rather more concrete situation than the previous one. But the continuum starts and ends at a higher abstract level than the vocational training or institutional care continua that are currently utilized.

This greater complexity and abstract quality to a continuum may explain why, in an historical sense, rehabilitation in home living skills started later. Another relevant aspect, also abstract in terms of historical development, has been the ideological shift arguing for integration of individuals into home-like community settings which, in its own right, has brought about a practical concern for more complex rehabilitation processes.

It appears that the introduction of tasks, in historical terms, is correlated with the amount of concrete and abstract content involved. If this is correct then we should be able to arrange projected tasks into a system of abstractness and complexity which should facilitate the design of a developmental hierarchy. This has training value, and would enable us to forecast which and when new procedures should become incorporated into a particular continuum.

Leisure and recreation training

The need for physical recreation has been recognized for a long period of time. However, the development of community recreation and leisure time activities as a part of the normal rehabilitation continuum is only just commencing. This involves a more abstract conception of rehabilitation because in temporal and relevancy terms this area seems more remote from direct rehabilitation than the other areas which have been discussed.

Many training staff do not understand the importance of leisure training. Beck-Ford et al. (1984) indicated through direct quotes the verbal attitudes of many staff, e.g. 'There is not time.' 'People should relax at home, they have had enough training.' Some staff indicated there were more important activities to carry out. Many leisure skills involve considerable abstract and temporally distant components which make it difficult for many trainers to recognize why such activities are necessary. They represent a method through which abstract and temporally remote skills can be developed. Many decision-making skills can be developed through leisure time. This is critical if the individual is to function responsibly within society.

Leisure time may be one of the most important areas in which training can be carried out because it occupies, and if current economic situations continue will occupy, much of the person's waking day. As such it then makes up the greater part of programme structure, and can come to represent one of the major resources for rehabilitation. No less important is the fact the individual is interested in such activities and gains self-motivation and self-esteem from involvement with the projects themselves. Physical development, including muscle tone and body posture can be improved. All of these attributes have effect on a person's ability to obtain employment.

It is of interest that individuals quite frequently fail in the community because of inappropriate activity during their leisure hours. Without appropriate leisure time, either on one's own or with others, it is difficult for individuals to become involved in society. They become isolated and may fail. This failure may occur not only in home and local community performance, but in their vocational employment, since failure in employment is frequently caused by insurmountable difficulties in these areas. For example, late arrival for work or inappropriate emotional behaviour at work may be a direct result of fatigue, emotional outbursts or delinquent behaviour in other settings.

Even within the area of leisure time a range of concrete to abstract skills are found. Such a range of activities is clearly identified in the regular community by Nash (1953), who suggested a hierarchy of leisure time and recreational skills, based on observation of how individuals spend their leisure hours. The hierarchy of leisure activities involves four levels. The first level involves skills of an observational or non-participatory type. Individuals watch events—such as television or films. Little activity is required on their part; they are essentially passive observers of other people's activities. The second stage is one in which the individuals carry out largely non-participatory or simple activities with others. This level includes a wide range of simple social activities, e.g. having coffee with a friend, playing a simple game. Thus a social component is introduced which involves more diverse and competing stimulation.

The third stage involves participatory activities, but they are organized for the disabled person by others. Further, the events are generally of a gross physical nature, and are extremely important in terms of motor development. They are often carried out as a group process, e.g. swimming, football. Because of the important connection between motor activity and physiological health, such performance appears relevant to motivation level. It seems clear, if this hierarchy is accepted, that leisure activity is critical to effective development in other areas, but third-level attainment may be necessary before this component can influence the other areas very positively.

There is a fourth level where the individual is the organizer of leisure time; it is referred to as a creative or self-actualization level. The individual plans for future events and makes arrangements of a social nature, often involving other people. This type of co-ordination requires abstract skill including temporal judgement. The arrangements may be socially complex where meaningful communication involving time, place and equipment are essential. The individual must develop internal structures and organization patterns to do this successfully. When the individual masters this level he can function in a wide range of circumstances. This hierarchy has been confirmed by Beck, Possberg and Brown (1977) amongst mentally handicapped adults, and it has been further identified in children suffering from physical disabilities. Further support comes in a study by Brown, Hughson and Nemeth (1981), who examined leisure activities amongst disabled adults in a rural area. Recently, Brown (1986b) has conducted a leisure recreation survey amongst a small group of handicapped boys and girls in an Arab community. The same four levels apply with a lack of opportunities for leisure time at the more advanced phases.

Obviously within each of these levels there is a hierarchy of skills from simple to complex. Some involve no major social skills while others involve very important social communication skills. For example, it is much more likely that the complex problems of problem-solving will arise on a wilderness camp than when one is playing a simple game of cards. When severely retarded persons have been on wilderness camps, one major aspect of behaviour that has been noted is the wide range of skills that such individuals can demonstrate (Hughson, Berrien and Brown, 1978). The same supervisors who had worked with the individuals the rest of the year had not noticed these skills on previous occasions. A new and challenging situation, if appropriately controlled, is likely to bring out resources which have not been seen in the disabled individual. The same phenomenon has been noted in learning-disabled children who after three weeks of camping show advances in educational aspects of behaviour (Samuels, 1985).

Leisure skills also provide opportunities to teach a wide range of skills that are needed for effective performance in other areas of people's lives. Indeed none of these are really separate when it comes to functioning. Individuals who have advanced leisure time skills may proceed to higher levels in other areas of performance, although some variation between the continua or areas is likely. For example, independence is more likely to be found in vocational than home living skills simply because the tasks generally involve a higher degree of structure.

Behaviour in disabled persons is believed to follow the basic developmental patterns of normal individuals. Thus any rehabilitation process should follow such a sequence. This is probably fairly well accepted in children's basic motor skills, but the evidence in this section demonstrates quite clearly the similarity between hierarchical development of skills in normal and disabled persons. The data from Nash (1953) and Mundy (1976) with normal persons very closely follows that of Beck et al. (1977) with disabled individuals, except the disabled persons show, for the most part, greater restriction in leisure skills and are forced massively to over-learn the less complex skills. Thus they are once again in double jeopardy—they are taught to learn and perseverate at a low level of operation, without opportunity or training to deal with the higher-level activities, which can lead to the diversified performance and improved concept attainment which is relevant to vocational, home living and other areas. Again transfer is inhibited, not because the individual cannot do the task which represents his ability to transfer, but because there are barriers to demonstrating the new skill. Agencies which only provide vocational training are very restricted, and place their clients at a great disadvantage. Leisure training, because of its complex social nature at community levels, is ideal for the training of transfer, partly because a combination of learnt skills is required. For example, if an individual decides that she would like to go on a picnic with a friend, and has received adequate training in this area, then it is likely that she will have: (a) travel skills, (b) money-handling skills, and (c) social and communication interaction skills, as well as (d) a wide range of motor skills. However, there are also planning skills involving preparation. Time sequencing over short and long periods becomes necessary. In these circumstances the practitioner begins to teach advanced-level skills of operation in an abstract mode. Obviously many individuals are not at the advanced level indicated by this example, yet at each stage of the leisure time training continuum, appropriate skills are available to teach individuals in a stepwise fashion from the simple to complex levels.

It is understandable, historically, that leisure time training should occur last, so most agencies have not yet begun to train skills in leisure time activities as part of a training regime. Very often they expose individuals to leisure time without providing the necessary training. Task analysis and the development of a hierarchy of training procedures in the leisure time area were virtually nonexistent until the mid-1980s (Beck-Ford *et al.*, 1984; Levine *et al.*, 1984). Furthermore, it is extremely difficult to obtain funds for leisure time training, partly because government offices do not see the relevance of such activities as a fundamental of rehabilitation. Perhaps, more accurately, those government offices concerned with social services perceive leisure funding as the responsibility of some other ministry, so it becomes difficult, politically, to argue *who* is responsible or interested. Governments can hardly be blamed for this view when most of the rehabilitation profession do not bring the need clearly to the fore. The scientific community appears less interested in leisure time activities as they relate to the rehabilitation field than other features of disability. One simple example is that of the 1979 meeting of the International Congress for the Scientific Study of Mental Retardation, which produced only one paper on leisure rehabilitation amongst the many hundreds of papers presented. Yet greater sensitivity is emerging. In 1984 at least six books were published dedicated to leisure time training for handicapped persons.

Leisure training is a good example of lack of development of rehabilitation philosophy and technical structure of programmes. It may, of course, be argued that in certain types of physical ailment, e.g. heart disease, physical recreation is prescribed, but this merely serves to underline the present argument. Practitioners recognize concrete physical activities as important prior to any understanding of the need for more abstract activities. For example mental recreation in the form of problem-solving games may be highly therapeutic in certain types of central nervous systems deterioration. Secondly, leisure activity is seen as physical and recreational rather than physical, social or psychological, and the leisure component is not perceived as the essential characteristic.

The need for a leisure training continuum can be made for ageing populations (Palmore, 1980) where the stimulating qualities of leisure activities, such as games that the individual has traditionally enjoyed, may help to maintain or reactivate problem-solving abilities, motivation and physical fitness. Yet frequently the games employed in units for so-called geriatric populations are simple group activities often chosen by the staff. The importance of individual choice, awareness of the individual's prior leisure interests and acceptance of activities may often be overlooked. For example, an elderly man whose leisure passion was gardening might be provided with activities relating to plants, yet the upkeep of plants is often the responsibility of staff members within an agency. The clients become non-participatory observers—i.e. level 1 in the hierarchy described! The above represents a common example of what might be termed activity substitution. Staff know that flowers are appreciated and therefore they are supplied. The activities of planting, tending and caring—which constitute, for many, much of the pleasure—are denied.

Sometimes care-givers recognize the need, but not the process. For example, Brown, Bayer and MacFarlane (1985) found that mentally handicapped adults, whose parents or sponsors recognized the need for friendship, often promoted contact with others by encouraging visitors. But the friendship was often of a non-participatory type, and after acknowledgement and greeting had taken place further interaction occurred through communication between non-handicapped adults. In such circumstances there needs to be a redirection of attention, a clear recognition of purpose and planning of communication. This may interfere with the final object of casual and informal social meetings. But initially training in social interaction has to be structured (Brown, Bayer and MacFarlane, 1986).

If we can carry out training in the leisure time area we can teach many of the concrete and abstract skills that are necessary for functioning effectively within society. Given that individuals gain such skills it is likely that they will become more accepted by relatives, friends and the rest of the community. However, there are other aspects that are important in this context.

Employment, society and leisure

Given the current times of economic restraint, it is unlikely that employment is going to be available for many disabled persons in our community. Further, it is somewhat doubtful whether the rather positive economic climate in the 1970s will be repeated for non-handicapped individuals, let alone the handicapped members of our community. Thus a major change in lifestyle is forecast. This has relevance to rehabilitation priorities and therefore programmes. Historically what has happened is understandable. But it must be asked whether it is wise to persevere in the development of essentially vocational agencies and continue with largely vocational routines within the rehabilitation domain. Work training is easy, straightforward, it keeps people occupied, it provides concrete tasks, and it is easy to administer. However, if the traditional concepts and procedures of rehabilitation are to be challenged and the anticipated reversal to reinstitutionalization averted (Brown, 1984b), it is necessary to have a new and effective philosophy, together with the technology to put it into effect.

This immediately raises questions concerning the suggested trend towards reinstitutionalization. Many staff recognize that individuals who would once have been brought into agencies in the community, or would have been rehabilitated to the community, are being returned or maintained within larger institutions. This does not mean that there is no movement of clients from institutions into the community, but rather that efforts in the opposite direction are again occurring. In some Canadian communities individuals are being sent to new types of institutions in rural areas, and a major reason for this relates to the desire to provide adequate employment to normal citizens in non-industrial areas and non-urban communities. Handicapped people can be moved to these rural areas and thus by their presence provide local people with jobs. This process is likely to accelerate as individuals without jobs turn increasingly to criminal or other antisocial activities. More reasons for institutionalizing people, and more ways to institutionalize and economically house large groups of 'deviant' people, will arise. Once the cycle begins it becomes reinforced by other social, economic and environmental variables. As Mitchell (1986) points out, the family with a handicapped child is influenced by a variety of environmental levels which are interrelated. But the system is mutually interdependent. Thus disabled persons influence their surrounding environment—sometimes positively and at other times negatively. The same behaviour at one period will meet with a compassionate response, but at other times will be rewarded with a response which is negative to the individual but serving other goals in the community. Rehabilitation personnel, governments, disabled people themselves, and relatives and friends must understand this complex interaction if they are to come to control the system. An understanding of the processes outlined above is relevant, if not fundamental, to this requirement.

If the range of lifestyles for disabled persons are changed by providing structured skill training for leisure pursuits it will be possible to provide options for non-work activities which might minimize the trends listed above. But this calls for a major change in Western society's thinking which, to this point, has preserved and rewarded a puritan work ethic (Toffler, 1980). Society now faces a problem where many individuals, including handicapped persons, need to behave effectively in terms of non-work time if they are to maintain or obtain roles as functional and valued members of society. It is not suggested that people should not learn work skills; on the other hand it is believed that the singular accent on vocational rehabilitation neither does service to the disabled person nor is it consistent with society's behavioural goals. The social and non-work skills are the very ones that are needed most, and are invariably used when individuals live effectively in their local community with normal peers.

Critical examination of the continua

At this stage it is important to examine each of the programme continua for training in rather more detail. As indicated earlier four major continua are proposed—vocational, social education, home living and leisure training. The vocational continuum runs from basic orientation and introduction of vocational training to concrete work skills. An individual may have to be trained prior to this point in such areas as attention to task and gross motor skills. Basic work skills, such as implementing one- or two-step verbal or visual instructions which require only two or three movements, and an ability to maintain specific behaviours, consistently repeated over time to complete a task, form the basic components for the first stage of structured vocational training. A more advanced stage is the application of work routines and the demonstration of acceptable interpersonal skills with other workers, all of which are best taught in actual or simulated vocational environments. This is followed by a preplacement intervention phase with opportunities for work experience in the community and finally, placement in job trial (Marlett and Hughson, 1977; Brown and Hughson, 1980; Whelan and Speake, 1981). Another approach is the application of the non-facility-based supported work model. For example Brown *et al.*'s (1985) research indicates early functional training of young children with severe handicaps can result in stable job placement in community settings without periods of training in vocational agencies. Nevertheless the characteristics of structured and long-term training are still present.

A clearer continuum would be formed if vocational skills were purely as defined and did not include those of a social nature. We might regard this area as 'basic movement and assembly processes' and conceive of it running from basic attentional and motor tasks through to performance on work situations. In using such a modified continuum it becomes apparent, as one progresses to the upper end of the continuum, that opportunities for group rather than individual work become available, and opportunities for work in the community with supports are also possibilities as out-reach components (McCarthy, 1984). It is quite clear that as one proceeds along this continuum, it moves into a stage where it intermeshes with other areas such as social and educational learning (see Figure 4). It should be borne in mind that social skills must be taught in the vocational milieu in an integrated fashion, and equivalent social skills also need to be taught in community and home living environments (e.g. taking directions, dressing appropriately, arriving on time to social events and meeting friends). This involves both specific learning and transfer.

Structured training and performance alone are insufficient for rehabilitation. External, formalized, environmental structures must be replaced by internalized processes. If people (parents, supervisory staff) are not going to be present to help the individual decide and perform, or tasks are to be taught that are not so routine, the individual must know what to do in a particular instance and be able to perform adequately. The assembly steps in the manufacture of a simple electronic switching gear can be analysed and presented in a very clear-cut sequence. Thus the task can be structured and its performance supervised within a work environment. However an individual who is required to catch a bus to travel from place A to place B may face a variety of circumstances. It may be raining at the bus stop, there may be a crowd so that the individual is unable to get on the bus, he or she might have the wrong change, or sit next to somebody who asks questions that cannot be dealt with. The point is that some aspects of task learning in static situations can be concretized or structured, but once variations emerge, with consequent varied responses, it is not possible to rely on structured learning alone. One cannot ensure staff are present all the time to deal with continual variations in the situation.

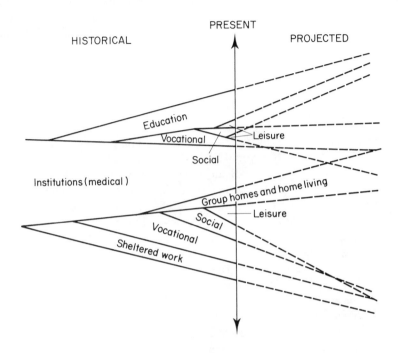

Figure 4. Development of integrated rehabilitation programmes over time.

Task training may commence with structured learning, but in the end plans must be made for the individual to learn to make his or her own response selections. This is unstructured performance where the controls lie with the individual. The aim is gradually to remove external structure so that the individual can still function effectively within an increasingly unstructured situation.

It is interesting that it appears there is a hierarchy in terms of structures that have been created in the programmes delivered by staff in the field of mental handicap. Vocational rehabilitation is a relatively highly structured performance compared with social or community rehabilitation. Yet within each of these dimensions there is a continuum from high to low structure in learning and performance. A more advanced domain is the area of home living skills, which tends to take place over long periods of time, but often involves fairly unstructured situations. Finally there are the leisure time skills which are very open-ended, and a personalized internal structure is frequently required. Of course these systems overlap, and within each one of them there is a dimension from structure to lack of structure or open-ended environmental decision-making.

It is important to recognize that individuals who attend any rehabilitation programme vary in the levels at which they start within the different continua. As noted elsewhere, it is important to obtain a baseline in terms of each individual's behaviour and commence training from that level. As skills are integrated across continua (a process often ignored in practice), multiple baselines provide the information for further training. Individuals, may for example, perform well vocationally and be very ineffective in home living skills. The obverse can happen, but is less likely to occur because of the relatively advanced nature of the home living continuum.

The problems of transfer from one continuum area to another are important, and of course progress is impeded or advanced by attitudes of personnel in the different rehabilitation environments. These often give rise to major problems in the rehabilitation process. Staff operating a vocational programme in a positive direction may be thwarted, for example, by negative attitudes within the home living situation. Alternatively, training staff may implement different and conflicting training models in the different areas. Disabled individuals are sometimes required to learn from two antithetical systems compared with the normal individual who may only be required to adapt to one. Perhaps more importantly, developmentally normal individuals take information and build it into their own repertoire in their own way, thus adapting it to their own learning style. This is often not possible for individuals who are disabled and yet, in turn, they may have imposed on them conflicting learning formats. One of the values of continua description is that it encourages the development of systematic and integrated programming relevant to individual needs.

Social education is often seen as a range of particular skills which, on closer analysis, divides into two major areas. Community survival skills such as social sight reading vocabulary, basic arithmetical skills, number recognition and budgeting skills are a constellation of competencies to be developed. Training is also necessary in social skills which are required for the development of satisfying interpersonal relationships. The original continuum put forward earlier is not homogeneous, and in one sense is not a true continuum. We now need a further model for interpersonal—social skill training (Rosen, Clark, and Kivitz, 1977; Johnson, 1984).

In the leisure time area some of the basic skills, starting with observation and non-participatory types of activity, have already been noted. But it is also important to ensure that physical education develops appropriately. The early part of any continuum consists of basic programme skills, and this is true of leisure time and recreation skills.

Individuals, through exposure to and involvement with activities, may become interested in a range of different forms of games and recreation interests. However, such interests are unlikely to develop unless individuals are required to participate in a number of activities in the first instance. Contemporary concern for human rights often overlooks the fact that most people do not gain interests by mere exposure to activities. Many gain interest because they are required to carry out activities. Familiarity and success results in enjoyment and reward in particular activities and skills, and motivation often increases because there are opportunities for success in situations which the individual may not have initially selected for himself. In this sense there is a form or structure to the initial programme. If the individual gradually shows signs of interest in particular activities, specific skills can be developed. It is important that such interests are not just limited to organized games because the aim is to encourage individuals to become 'self-starters' in a variety of leisure time activities. Mere exposure to community recreation is insufficient. The individual needs to learn the basic skills involved in active leisure participation.

This structured approach may be an anathema to those who believe in freedom of choice, yet they must remember that choice comes from knowledge and experience. On the other hand, to ensure the approach is not simply arbitrary or authoritarian, the practitioners involved must have a clear and knowledgeable professional philosophy and be sufficiently versatile that they can change requirement to choice and vice-versa as need arises. In terms of rehabilitation this is one of the areas where little progress has been made.

Many skills in the other continua integrate with leisure time activities. In order for an individual progressively to acquire competent community leisure skills successfully, the individual must gain certain basic skills in the other areas. Certain social education skills have to be learned and applied; for example, learning to ride the bus in order to go to the cinema. The requirement for the integration of skills produces a conceptual leisure time continuum, which is more involved and complex than some of the other areas. Unfortunately once individuals leave a vocational training setting, other necessary social skills may not be taught, and individuals are expected to learn social skills by themselves. Many agencies or services stop the rehabilitation process when an individual is vocationally 'placed' or is living relatively independently. Rehabilitation does not work this way. Training may be complete in a particular area but must be continued in other areas. In the above model rehabilitation is a continuous and never-ending process.

Eventually individuals should be able to make their own arrangements for leisure, which will mean that they can spontaneously arrange for their own specific leisure time activities and can do them on a regular basis. They will be able to communicate with friends, and set up and follow through with the leisure activities. Of course, any individual may plateau at any stage within the continuum. If this occurs the individual cannot fully control his or her own environment. In such cases it is necessary to ensure that staff remain involved in the continuation and maintenance of a supportive structure for the individual—in other words, maintained semi-dependence. This should be seen as effective rehabilitation, but it must be done in such a way that staff recognize when the individual is again ready to progress. Plateaus in development are common—continuous unbroken progress is not! This is an aspect of training which has been given little attention over the years, for it is thought that once individuals are in the community they can function effectively. Indeed, as systems change in the community even individuals who have become self-supporting regress and often get into difficulties. Transit systems may change, shops may close, and habits which are familiar to the disabled person may no longer be useful. They then have to learn new behaviours.

The same concerns arise in all areas of disability where the individual is deprived of community involvement. For example the mentally ill person who requires a period of hospitalization and the physical traumatized individual who has been 'out of community circulation' have difficulties in adapting and relearning once they re-enter a community. The fact that sometimes a different community is employed from their traditional home base makes the problem more complex. Means of dealing with problems of unfamiliarity or refamiliarization are dealt with in a subsequent chapter. Under such circumstances it becomes important to encourage community involvement by agency staff. Informal networks of people who can support and plug gaps in experience are necessary.

Models of rehabilitation

It can be seen from Figure 4 that expansion in service areas and the proliferation of the dimensions of service can provide major conflict in the areas of programming and jurisdiction. Concerns may arise in a variety of areas. There may be the development of discrete services which may not relate one to another. The expansion provides opportunities for disruption and breakdown of services across the different areas. Finally, it accounts for the development of a variety of new services from different areas. For example social education has developed from both hospital and school systems. This has the advantage of different interests and models, and the disadvantage of negative competition and confusing and competing directions to service.

Such a model provides an opportunity to ask what further types of programmes are likely to develop. The model suggests areas of greater complexity, greater community involvement and interdependent staffing needs. One possible area is that of spiritual needs of individuals who are handicapped. This implies progress in addressing the internal needs of clients associated with people's quality of life and higher-order needs. Staff will be obliged to further the development of the individual's unique cultural, social and religious or spiritual background, and to enable the individual to find expression within his or her own cultural milieu. There is still a marked tendency in rehabilitating individuals to strive for middle-class standards of living, which sometimes excludes persons from the rehabilitation process (e.g. emotionally disturbed persons, those in conflict with the law).

The model also suggests that there may be a move to greater community involvement and a recognition that the various training needs should be co-ordinated. However, this supposes three requirements: (1) that rehabilitation can take place in the community, in which case there will be a reduction of formal training environments, a move which would be consistent with a decline in vocational training; (2) that quality of life can be preserved or enhanced, which presupposes an adequate monitoring and advocacy system; and (3) that there will be a recognition of individual variability and needs so that selection of appropriate programmes and programme plans becomes possible. All three of these requirements are currently developing.

In highlighting vocational programming it is of some interest that it is in rural areas that the first flush of community individualization of employment is becoming successful. It is speculated that this may be related to the lack of bureaucracy typical of the large urban agencies. The growth of advocacy, the training of rehabilitation practitioners (see later chapter), and the development of IPP (individual programme plans), along with service brokerage, all seem consistent with such developments.

Concluding comments

An attempt has been made to chart the progress of rehabilitation primarily in the field of mental handicap, from institutionalization to community integration. It has been argued that the development of services can be seen as certain continua which follow a concrete to abstract formulation and relate to the nature of our processes of discovery. Yet these continua represent steps in a rehabilitation process and the appropriateness of different stages needs to be examined for its current rehabilitation value. As social circumstances change, so do rehabilitation needs. Thus not only is rehabilitation a continuous process, it is also a continually changing process which nevertheless follows basic principles. Within this process, individual needs must be met. Integration and consistency across the various continua are essential, though progress by an individual within different areas may vary.

The conceptual model put forward seems representative of that of other areas of disability, though development in other areas may be more or less advanced. For example, institutional care is still a major practice in the field of criminality and is still extensive in mental illness, and geriatrics. The recent study of Segger and Plecas (1987) demonstrates the applicability of the social education continuum for institutionalized offenders. Thus developmental steps or continua described here could be helpful in examining and providing services in all areas of disability.

The history of our own development of rehabilitation services is the history of development of an individual's cycle of learning. It is understandable and necessary that we start with large institutions; that we come to develop vocational training programmes; and that, in the end, we move to more elaborate and abstract forms of service. It is necessary because of our personal knowledge and allied cognitive constructs; it is also necessary because of the type of training that we can give personnel. It is rarely argued, yet is probably true, that one of the reasons that we have required structures for the delivery of service in the past is because of the low level of training of staff. Without effective training a need is seen to mass staff together in hierarchical structures in order to control the services that they deliver. In many cases training is essentially provided at a care-giving level with attempts to protect rather than encourage the development of new behaviour.

CHAPTER FOUR

An integrated model of behavioural rehabilitation

Introduction

In order to build a model of rehabilitation it is necessary to recognize that behaviour occurs in a variety of dimensions which interact with each other over time. Unfortunately this is often not appreciated in traditional rehabilitation situations. In this chapter an attempt is made to collect several of the arguments and descriptions in earlier chapters, together with information relating to a range of behavioural processes employed in rehabilitation settings. The consolidation of training continua (e.g. vocational and social education), with the need for structure in the learning process, is examined in relation to a range of behavioural phenomena.

It is important to recognize that there are a number of dimensions or areas of learning which interface with one another. In this case we are referring to the various programme areas which are loosely defined and described within various community agencies. There is also a dimension which can be labelled the history of programming, and this can not only help us understand why certain programmes run in particular ways, but also assist in projecting the development of programmes in a coherent and predictable manner.

This chapter is concerned with the development of these areas of knowledge and, from their integration, the types of behavioural strategies which are important for specific individuals can be deduced. The chapter represents an attempt to provide a model which will enable the trainer or teacher to perceive the interlocking nature of various dimensions of rehabilitation. The ultimate aim is to produce a coherent philosophy of rehabilitation, an effective training structure for specific individuals, and a means of generating an effective organization model for rehabilitation service delivery.

Rehabilitation as a process over time

Where instructors have been taught task analysis and individual programme planning, the longer-term implications of training are often overlooked. As a result an individual may be taught a task effectively, but not retain a high performance level over time because the skill is not integrated into the overall programme training matrix. For example, in work by Hughson, Berrien and Brown (1978) a series of task analyses were developed for individuals working in a pre-vocational unit. Although the individuals were severely handicapped, many of them learned a wide range of specific tasks and eventually, because of the increase in their baseline level of performance, were moved to more formal vocational settings. In this study individuals were followed over a period of time, and it was found that many of the skills which had been learned were not retained six months later. Analysis of the programmes in the particular workshops attended showed that the tasks were never used or practised in the workshops, and therefore there were no opportunities for the individuals to employ their previously learned skills.

In many areas of disability a range of curriculum packages have been developed, but the lack of recognition for the need to integrate these packages into the overall programme and their relevance over time is one of the major limitations in effective rehabilitation. This becomes increasingly important as curriculum packages cover a wider range of performance domains (Johnson-Martin, Jens and Attermeier, 1986).

Children frequently rehearse previously learned tasks in normal learning and use them as building blocks for subsequent learning. Thus frequent repetition of a story or repetition of a skill learned on a tricycle can be generalized to other situations. Under these circumstances individuals do not tend to lose the original skills. In disabled persons such attainment may have to be formally planned and stimulated by the trainer. It is critical that opportunities for the integration of such learning are provided, and that there is formal understanding of such a learning matrix in the application of training programmes. But this requires that practitioners also recognize precisely what it is that the individual needs and will be able to use in his environment as he moves from one stage to another in the rehabilitation process.

Human learning generally proceeds by very specific and organized steps. When there is a disability this guideline is even more critical. There are two elements to be borne in mind: firstly, the profile and the sequence of skill-building over time (rate of development) and secondly, an element that can be referred to as teaching structure. This, too, has a profile and an historical sequence.

There are two aspects to teaching structure: (1) informal structure or general background structure in terms of physical and social dimensions, and (2) formal teaching structure. Time is seen as (a) personal time, i.e. what happens to an individual during his lifespan; and (b) historical time, which relates to occurrence of events over any long time period, normally longer than the individual's life span, such as accumulation of knowledge.

Individual and programme interaction—concerns relating to implementation

It is necessary to look at programming over time, and this is true of all rehabilitation dimensions that have been introduced. The behaviour that individuals show relates to their own development in time through maturation and general experience, but it also relates to them in terms of the impact of special programmes they experience over time. At any particular phase of development the individual will not necessarily show the same behaviour as at another time; nor is he or she expected to show the same behaviour in different programmes at the same point in time. This has relevance to specific programme development, goal-setting, application of learning principles and the employment of specific programme material and apparatus. But these attributes are often absent and training needs of the client are frequently overlooked. We have observed this in a wide range of agencies in a number of countries. For example personnel in agencies may purchase or design apparatus or a programme curriculum which is demonstrated to be effective. But as soon as apparatus breaks down, or the designer or purchaser leaves, it is relegated to a storeroom or to a cupboard and is not employed again. The fact that programme material can be put on one side illustrates that, in rehabilitation, an understanding of the need for formal integration of hierarchies within a knowledge system—i.e. that particular tools, apparatus, curriculum materials are required at specific points in time—has not yet developed.

The fundamental philosophical concepts that training is based on sequence, and that people, however handicapped, can learn, do not seem to be part of the accepted beliefs of staff in a wide range of units for disabled persons. Rehabilitation units are frequently viewed as places where people are 'stored' and given some activities to make them happy. There is often little recognition of the fact that disabled persons can learn effectively and will be able to adapt to a wide range of situations provided learning is given in a sequence-wise fashion. Even the accepted philosophy of normalization appears bereft of adequate technical support systems, and in recent investigations it has been shown (Brown, Bayer and MacFarlane, 1985) that although an agency may forward a mission statement which encompasses normalization and integration of disabled persons into the community, it frequently does not practise the philosophy. For example in five vocational rehabilitation agencies in Western Canada examined by Brown *et al.* (1985), the placement rate from training to work placement in a 12-month period was under two per cent, and individuals who had been at the agencies for a period of five years had a zero placement rate in the sixth year. Individuals may be moved from large institutions, but institutionalization can and does occur in other settings!

The problem at the everyday level of practice comes in many forms and at all levels. For example, in an agency within a developing country, children were taught to ride bicycles. But the bicycles eventually broke down. Staff did not know how to repair them so they were put into storage. Breakdown of the mechanical device caused a lack of further training. The same situation also applies in a wide range of rehabilitation situations in homes for elderly people when television sets do not work effectively, in the recreation field where materials or apparatus break down and in normalization environments when there are insufficient group homes. These instances relegate rehabilitation to a storage system or, if placement is insisted upon, merely represent a dumping process in the community. If rehabilitation is to be effective then the necessary programme stages, and the necessary apparatus, are all required and must be formally in operation. No-one would tolerate a surgical procedure where the apparatus used in anaesthesia broke down and could not be employed. Once again we recognize the situation is unacceptable when it is concrete and traumatic or when it is physically related to most human beings (i.e. 'us'). We have not reached the point where this type of professional concern and expertise is regularly, formally and frequently available in agencies dealing with behavioural and social rehabilitation.

Learning principles

In order to understand the rehabilitation process more clearly it is necessary to look at the variety of learning or training principles which make up each of its dimensions. Probably the first principle to investigate relates to the individual; the internal processes which affect the particular learning and performance he or she shows at any particular point in time. Human learning is believed to proceed by particular rules, and, in a very real sense, the impact of these processes is more easily observed in any individual when he is involved in new and original learning. Although new or original learning is generally observed in young individuals, it is more readily and more continuously apparent when an individual suffers from a handicap. Learning is then particularly slow, and it is difficult for a person to master skills. Other individuals, of the same age, who have no handicap, master the same skills relatively easily and quickly. But the situation is more complex than this. The disabled individual is often at a much earlier stage of learning than the normal person. He thus spends more time in a state of early learning. Early learning is seen to be slower in the handicapped person than in the average person. The phenomenon is not only true of individuals who are disabled at birth but includes persons who have recently gained their handicaps. The latter persons are suddenly thrust into an early learning mode. They will behave to some degree like new learners and thus will show a range of behaviours that are described here. However the presentation of their behaviour may be more complex than that of individuals handicapped from birth, partly because of uneven and differential handicap, including personal knowledge of their pre-handicap behaviour which has emotional and self-image connotations.

What are some of the attributes of early behaviour and learning? First of all, when individuals are confronted with new tasks they require very frequent and considerable stimulation in order to learn effectively. The stimuli have to be frequently repeated and response bonds have to be gradually strengthened. Once the individual has started to respond appropriately to stimulation he/she tends to over-generalize responses to other situations, partly because of the perceived similarity of stimulation. This inappropriate responding has to be restricted so that the individual only applies knowledge or skill in the appropriate situation. A direct consequence of the above is that early learning is very slow, and at times appears to involve major error in the form of over-generalization, which in reality is part of the normal cycle of the learning process. It may be inferred that learning is likely to increase in rate and range over time as early learned skills are applied to new situations.

Already in these few brief sentences it has been indicated that there are a number of dimensions to the learning process. Stimuli need to be repeated frequently but as people 'learn how to learn' fewer repetitions are required. Learning starts very slowly. Learning passes from over-generalization to restriction of responses in appropriate situations. Thus a dimension or continuum exists in which learning improves as more and more tasks are learned and transfer processes gradually speed up.

However, within the process of learning there is another phenomenon which should be introduced. Learning tends to be cyclic. This must be borne in mind when we examine behaviour, and particularly learning amongst handicapped persons. As individuals proceed to attack new learning situations, behaviour which has recently been established will tend to show regression. This is likely to occur each time a new learning situation is introduced. Thus individuals will constantly make advances followed by apparent regressions of behaviour. Lovaas (1966), for example, demonstrated that when autistic children first gained knowledge of words or sound combinations the introduction of further words or sound combinations caused a lowering of performance or forgetting of material which had recently been learned. The relearning of the initial material is more rapid on subsequent occasions and gradually regression or information loss is removed as other new information is introduced. Unfortunately the implications of this are often not applied in a consistent manner in rehabilitation. There are a number of phenomena of this kind. These should be borne in mind when constructing any remedial programme

Some of the dimensions or principles of learning appear to be important in promoting learning, and have major relevance for the design and application of programmes. It may be worth describing some of these principles in detail, for they are often not taken into account in the development of programmes.

Dimensions or principles of learning

Familiarity and unfamiliarity

The first dimension relates to the nature of familiarity and unfamiliarity. It relates not only to the unfamiliarity of the environment, but to the degree of familiarity of stimulation within a learning task. The phenomenon applies not only to the rehabilitation client but also to the technical and professional staff who are teaching handicapped persons.

Let us first consider the situation where the environment is unfamiliar. Figure 5 summarizes an experiment carried out by Brown and Semple (1970) where preschoolers, of about four years of age, were subjected to a change in physical and social stimulation. Children were required to carry out a simple task, namely to respond by naming parts of a doll which were pointed to by the experimenter. The experimenter was well known to the children who were seen in their 'home room' in the preschool. This is where the initial testing was also carried out. Following this initiation, half of the children continued each day in their classroom, while the remainder went to an adjacent, but relatively unfamiliar, room. The task remained the same throughout the testing period, as did the instructor. On the last assessment occasion the children switched groups so that those who had been tested in the classroom for several days were now in the unfamiliar environment, whereas those in the unfamiliar environment returned to their classroom. The experimental trials were of very short duration and thus the amount of time that each child was away from the familiar environment was very brief.

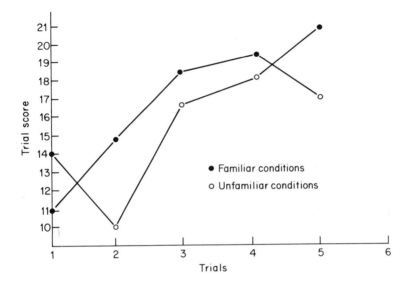

Figure 5. Language task mean score for two groups under familiar and unfamiliar conditions. (*Reproduced from Brown and Semple, 1970, with permission from* British Journal of Educational Psychology, *Scottish Academic Press, Edinburgh.*)

The results are quite clear. The number of words used by the children in the familiar situation gradually increased over the trials. This also applied to the children in the unfamiliar environment. But those in the unfamiliar environment used fewer words than the children in the familiar environment. When the conditions were reversed the children now in the unfamiliar environment showed a highly significant drop in their use of language.

The same phenomenon was seen when non-verbal behaviours were examined in familiar and unfamiliar environments. Non-verbal behaviour included motor movement relating to task performance, stereotype movement and global gazing. The amount and accuracy of movement was reduced in the unfamiliar environment, but global gazing and stereotyped behaviour increased.

The same phenomena have also been recorded by Brown (1965) working with older but handicapped children, and this is apparently consistent with the work of Hutt, Hutt and Ounstead (1965), who examined play behaviour in different disabled groups of young children with familiar and unfamiliar persons present. It seems that unfamiliar physical environments or unfamiliar people (social environments) reduce the amount of overt behaviour shown by children over a considerable time period.

Even well-established performance can be inhibited when unfamiliarity is introduced.

This leads to a number of important implications. It is recognized that most children or adults show an immediate decrement in performance when introduced to unfamiliar stimulation. Although adaptation may gradually occur, the effects can be traced for a considerable period of time. Further, if unfamiliarity is introduced into a situation there is a dramatic reduction in the amount of behaviour, even when the tasks or persons with the client are well known to the individual. The effect is also known to be dramatic when the individual is attempting to learn new material.

It would be wise to take such phenomena into account in a wide range of situations where people are required to learn or perform. Readers may be concerned about the generalizability of the data. For our part we are willing to take the risk that it applies as a reasonably reliable guideline in behaviour or as a blueprint of behaviour. There will, of course, be some variations. The work of Douglas and Blomfield (1949) indicates that very young children deprived of a mother figure, who have been hospitalized for a while, survive best in a familiar home environment rather than when removed to an unfamiliar environment with a substitute mother figure. The Prugh et al. (1953) study with children who were hospitalized is also relevant in this context. Some children had their mother present during their hospital stay and in other cases the mother was absent. Improvement was greatest amongst those children where some degree of contact with the mother figure was preserved. In other words where unfamiliarity is introduced it is important to keep other aspects of the social and physical environment familiar.

In the animal world there are a number of experiments involving the introduction of unfamiliar stimuli within familiar and unfamiliar environments (see Harlow, 1961). All of this information supports the generality of the rule that we are putting forward. It seems wise to take this knowledge into account in a wide range of situations where people are required to learn or perform. The phenomenon described seems greatest where new learning is involved, and the problem is further compounded when the individual is under stress or has a handicap. New learning requires a considerable degree of overt behaviour and our clinical impression is that the more handicapped the individual the more necessary it is for overt behaviour to occur hile learning takes place. Thus we predict increased inhibition with increase in degree of handicap, and therefore greatly impeded learning. In young but normal children overt behaviour is an important aspect of learning. Although it may not be a critical requirement for all learning, overt behaviour certainly seems to take place to a greater extent when highly original procedures or material are involved, or the child is very young. Youth and new learning are positively correlated.

We conclude that in order to learn effectively it is important that all aspects of the environment, including the learning situation, the materials and instructions, are familiar to the individual. If any feature of the situation is changed, behaviour is likely to be inhibited, at least for a brief period of time. The less well established the behaviour of an individual, the more likely that behaviour will be disturbed or inhibited by the introduction of unfamiliar stimuli.

Many disabled people find themselves in situations where they need to relearn a task. Trauma or chronic stress may mean that tasks once familiar and easily performed have been forgotten. Thus relearning needs to occur. The same familiarity-unfamiliarity principle applies. Disabled learners are frequently placed in situations where unfamiliarity occurs, and often show inhibition and distortion of behaviour. The problem is more complex than this because most handicapped persons have not experienced, during their early life, the range of unfamiliarity that is experienced by normal people. That is, due to slow learning or environmental protection, they do not have opportunities to explore new environments. Thus opportunities for learning how to learn are minimized. Handicapped persons thus become increasingly handicapped and more vulnerable than normal individuals.

During development the normal individual gradually learns to cope with unfamiliarity by trying out a range of unfamiliar situations. Although unfamiliar stimulation is threatening to the individual, he or she gradually gains greater control of such situations because of increasing experience. The person may still remain vulnerable to unfamiliarity under extreme circumstances. We may infer that any person who has not had a wide exposure to environmental stimulation or learning situations will show decrements of performance whenever confronted with unfamiliar stimuli. The decrements shown will be much greater than in the more experienced individual of similar age, who has learned to adapt, to some degree, to these circumstances.

It is reasonably apparent that a number of familiarization techniques could be readily introduced into rehabilitation programming to overcome some of the difficulties described. Although many readers may argue that the effects of unfamiliarity are obvious, our observations tell us that knowledge of this information is rarely taken into account in terms of the rehabilitation process.

It may be conjectured that unfamiliarity inhibits because of the startle nature of the stimuli, and the lack of any formulated plan to deal with the impact of the stimuli which come in unpredicted sequence. In a very real sense the individual cannot impose any plan on the situation, and therefore cannot respond appropriately. Unfamiliarity is thus a form of stress, and it is probably not inappropriate to generalize a model used to deal with unfamiliarity to stress situations, which by definition tend to be unfamiliar. Both appear to inhibit responses by the individual. One of the problems that confronts the new learner is that, in the very situation in which the individual needs to attempt new responses, he or she is likely to suffer inhibition and therefore produce fewer responses, and those that do occur will be of low intensity or even displaced.

Data that we are currently collecting suggest that some of the problems confronting non-readers, for example, may well result from a refusal to anticipate correct responses unless these are provided for them as models. In other words their lack of learning relates directly to the inhibition of overt responses, due to the lack of familiarity of the stimuli. Normal learners attempt to make responses more readily and therefore can benefit from feedback and more quickly experience reward.

The degree of familiarity is not just a quality of a stimulus in the environment, it is a quality of the stimulation in relation to the nervous system. Thus a stimulus not adequately processed because of central nervous system damage may appear to have a similar behavioural effect as a stimulus presented to a normal individual when that stimulus has not been presented previously. From a learning perspective the problem is much the same. In both instances the individual will need to receive the stimulus frequently if learning and adaptation are to take place.

Degree of familiarity is such an important variable, in terms of its effect, it might be conjectured that a wide range of unfamiliar stimuli presented at once, or few stimuli presented at high intensity, are likely to inhibit the learner because the degree of the unfamiliarity is increased. Some work by Hughson and Brown (1983) demonstrated that by doubling the number of instructional words presented to severely mentally handicapped learners, error rate was increased tenfold. This was not the case in mildly mentally handicapped persons. The results can be interpreted as an overload of information, but it is easier to overload information channels when stimulation is unfamiliar and therefore cannot be processed effectively. Therefore the greater the handicap the greater the possibility that stimuli will be regarded as unfamiliar.

A further attribute of unfamiliarity is that it tends to be meaningless, and cannot be readily interpreted. Once again there is a personal dimension for each individual, which runs from totally meaningless stimulation to meaningful stimulation. Unfamiliarity relates to a lack of interpretability of stimulation. Wide experience and ability to generalize will reduce meaninglessness and therefore the degree of unfamiliarity. Experience and the ability to generalize are associated with able learners and mature individuals, while mental disability, trauma, chronic and acute illness are associated with reduction of environmental experience, stress and increased meaninglessness of stimulation.

The implications are fairly apparent. The introduction of new information should be planned in advance. Students or clients should be trained or adapted to stimulation situations in terms both of environment and persons. Information should be introduced relatively quietly and should not be produced in great intensity or in great amount at any particular time. It should be presented slowly and repeated. As many dimensions as possible of a learning process should be kept familiar. Only one new dimension should be introduced at a time.

Some processes, because of their difficulty level, continue to be relatively unfamiliar or meaningless, and therefore it is important to recognize when elements in a total task are likely to appear unfamiliar to the individual. It has been observed in reading situations that where a word is not in an individual's reading vocabulary, not only is the individual unable to read this word, but he or she may have problems with the following words which have normally been within the person's reading vocabulary. The effects of meaninglessness, unfamiliarity and stress therefore generalize and increase the range of performance breakdown.

Language and rehabilitation

It has been noted elsewhere that young normal children can use language to control or improve motor behaviour. It has been demonstrated in a variety of experiments how this phenomenon takes place. It may well be that the importance of overt language in young children relates to attention properties, or that it provides a controlling mechanism for other behaviour. It can also act as a familiarization technique imparting meaning and precision to stimulation. The effects of this phenomenon are seen most clearly when we deal with non-verbal tasks and observe children's spontaneous language in dealing with such situations. It is believed that language is at first overt and becomes, with increasing use, covert in its format.

An interesting experiment carried out by Norrie (1970) dealt with language behaviour in junior and senior school children who were mentally handicapped, and were required to learn non-verbal tasks.

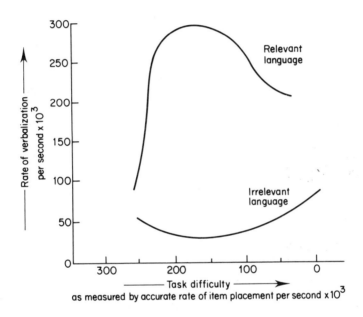

Figure 6. Verbalization and task difficulty. (Figure designed from data by Norrie, 1970.)

The tasks in this particular instance were a series of problems which required Lego blocks to be put together according to a specific format. The difficulty level of the tasks were first calibrated by examining the amount of time it took children to place items correctly. This is seen in the horizontal axis of the graph shown in Figure 6. The vertical axis shows the rate of verbalization or spontaneous language shown by the children. It is apparent that as the tasks increased in difficulty so there was a change not only in the amount of language produced, but also in the type of language which was omitted. The language was divided into two types: that which was relevant to the task in hand and that which was irrelevant. An example of relevant language was a series of words which described what the child was doing or wished to do in relation to the set task, such as 'I need a red one', 'I need to put it here'. Irrelevant language, on the other hand, was associated with comments apparently unrelated to the task in any meaningful way. Examples included language referring to events seen on television the previous evening. When the tasks were relatively simple, i.e. most children did them correctly, there was a considerable amount of irrelevant language. This reduced over the trials until approximately the 50/50 task pass-fail point was reached. After this point the amount of irrelevant language increased. The opposite occurred in the case of relevant language. Incidence was at first low but increased dramatically to the 50/50 pass-fail level, after which it gradually decreased. In other words, when learning was new but the task within the grasp of the children concerned, the language behaviour was related to the task, and presumably in some way assisted in the solving of the task at hand. When the task was easy, however, then the child did not need to be preoccupied with relevant language and could talk of other events. The individual could, in effect, do two tasks at the same time. We may also conjecture that when a task becomes too difficult a child begins to give up, and becomes more motivated and interested by other internal and external events or stimulation.

It might be interesting to speculate what happens if people are regularly presented with tasks which are too difficult for them. Using this model it would be predicted that individuals would produce a wide range of irrelevant language. In other words we would teach them how to be distractible or displace attention. Such behaviour may be regarded as highly emotional or disturbed behaviour. Although a task may be too difficult the individual still learns, but in this case is taught and learns how to be inappropriate! It is important to provide a task at the correct level of difficulty for that particular individual. The principle raises the hypothesis that handicapped or disturbed individuals, who are regularly asked to do tasks which are too difficult for them, are in fact trained to produce emotionally unstable forms of responding. If this is the case, at least in part, we may look at disturbance as a phenomenon induced by the trainer, teacher or supervisor, rather than anything that is intrinsically associated with abnormal pathology. The choice of appropriate tasks at the appropriate difficulty level becomes extremely important.

Generalization phenomena

Generalization is a major problem for a variety of handicapped persons. The results of experiments on generalization from learned responses are reasonably well known. They have been described in detail in the literature on animal behaviour and demonstrated in such tasks as the Lashley Jumping stand. Briefly, the problem is that the subject is given two stimuli which are reasonably identical. One requires a positive response, the other a negative response. Once the required responses have been learned the two stimuli which are on the same dimension (e.g. sound frequency) are moved closer together. The correct responses are still given since there is generalization of the responses to similar stimuli. If the two stimuli become sufficiently similar the subject is unable to distinguish between them. At this point behavioural breakdown occurs. Behaviour under these circumstances could be termed neurotic, but in one sense the responses are appropriate to a complex and difficult problem.

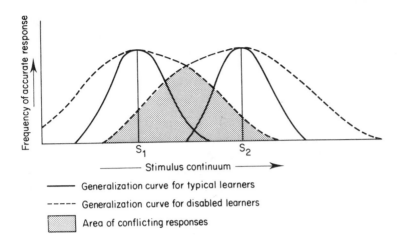

Figure 7. Schematic representation of generalization and early learning for typical and disabled learners.

In Figure 7, it is supposed that a handicapped individual has learned to respond to a particular stimulus in a particular fashion. To another stimulus the opposite response has been taught. Because of the difficulty that handicapped people have in discriminating stimuli of different types they reach the non-discrimination stage more rapidly than other persons. Furthermore, there is a tendency for over-generalization to occur once a particular stimulus has been learned. It may therefore be supposed, following the figure, that in the handicapped individual, unlike the normal learner, there is a much greater degree of overlap in terms of the area of 'not understanding' the response to make. This argues, in the first instance, for ensuring that stimuli which have opposite values are easily distinguished by the handicapped person concerned. This requires an individual decision for each client. The phenomenon is further highlighted by the work of Zeaman and House (1963), who posited that many handicapped learners have difficulty in discriminating correct stimuli from irrelevant stimuli. The accuracy of the responses in discrimination learning tend to be highly irregular and erratic for a long period of time during initial learning, particularly when compared with normal individuals. Fisher and Zeaman (1970) also note that there tends to be a breakdown in learning when a task is changed or becomes more difficult. This fits well with the concept of familiar and unfamiliar stimulation. What we are saying is that stimuli remain unfamiliar for much longer periods of time to handicapped individuals. It remains impossible for them to make the correct type of orienting responses to stimulation, for there is a long period of inappropriate or incorrect responding. We may also conjecture, having looked at the phenomenon of relevant and irrelevant language, that the chances of irrelevant language being produced by handicapped people is much higher than in non-handicapped people. This phenomenon will also last for a much longer period of time. The form of learning carried out by many handicapped people is likely to be slow, incorrect and frequently disturbed or displaced. Often it is regarded as inappropriate. It is necessary to consider whether they are learning inappropriate responses because we continually place them in inappropriate situations where they can only emit ineffective response patterns.

Motivation

We may well ask who is going to show the highest degree of responsiveness in any learning situation. The answer appears to be the person who shows a high level of motivation. Some work with disabled persons carried out by McKerracher *et al.* (1980) gives some support to this notion. However, although a reasonably linear relationship between motivation and the amount of responsiveness might be expected, a linear relationship between the amount of responsiveness and success would not be anticipated. If the individual finds it difficult to respond accurately, due to problems outlined above, displacement, including aggressive behaviour, may be emitted. Individuals of very low aggression tend to do rather poorly in rehabilitation situations, as do people of very high aggression. The most successful people appear to be individuals in the middle of the range, probably those who are slightly aggressive. In other words, aggressiveness (or possibly assertiveness), in some degree suggests that individuals are likely to produce responses at a level which enables them to learn from their environment.

Individuals who are over-responsive, particularly where there is a high error rate, are likely to be regarded as inappropriate within society, and because they produce such a wide range and large number of responses, are likely to be regarded as disturbed. In any case they are unlikely to process these responses effectively, and thus will be unable to relate positively and appropriately to their environment. Likewise individuals who show very low response rates do not provide sufficient response rates to modify behaviour, i.e. learn, and thus cannot begin to build up a wide repertoire of behaviour which we regard as normal and effective. They thus receive little reward from social interaction.

Stress and self-image

In Figure 8 three arrows are observed. The first represents increasing environmental stress and, as noted, environmental stress may be associated with a variety of phenomena such as unfamiliarity, meaningless stimuli, threat situations and new tasks. The second arrow in the reverse direction represents decreasing positive self-image. It is hypothesized that as individuals face rising environmental stress so their self-image decreases. Little is known about the interrelationship of these two phenomena, but common observation suggests that decrease in self-image is associated with environmental stress, and under these circumstances individuals are unable to produce their usual level of effective responding. For example, behaviour during hospitalization, of physically ill individuals who are otherwise normal, demonstrates the loss of self-image in relation to the environment.

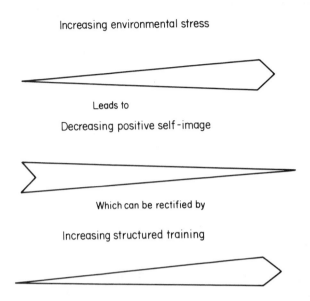

Increasing environmental stress

Leads to

Decreasing positive self-image

Which can be rectified by

Increasing structured training

Figure 8. Suggested relation between dynamic change in self-perception and environmental stress controlled by training structure.

The phenomenon of reduced self-image is interesting, particularly because a number of research workers have recently used this concept to describe aspects of handicap. Stott (1977) has pointed out that a high level of responding may be expected from handicapped children if they are in environments where they feel at ease and not under stress. Why, he asks, do so many handicapped children appear mentally handicapped in adult company, including teachers and parents, but when at play show a much higher level of appropriate responding? Feuerstein (1979), too, has suggested that mental handicap is more a phenomenon of one's knowledge about problem-solving than it is a phenomenon about basic lack of intelligence. The nature of self-image, its negative and positive aspects, need to be explored in much greater detail.

Structure of environment

If increasing environmental stress occurs, and this is associated with greater inability to respond appropriately, the following question arises. What changes in the environment or in the individual's circumstances would be required to bring about a rise in performance to approximate the individual's optimal response accuracy and rate of performance? One suggestion is that there needs to be increased structuring of the environment. When an individual can no longer cope with a situation, external signs and signals have to act as 'guide ropes'. They should direct the individual to appropriate responses. Another way of looking at this is to suggest that learning or performance has to become more overt and standardized, and aids or supports must be provided in the environment to bring this about. The individuals may produce some of these structures themselves. For example, they may start using overt language in relation to motor skills, or will increase the amount of familiarity, or demonstrate they can be successful in much simpler tasks where they still have sufficient positive self-image that they can produce appropriate behaviour.

The stress situations referred to are commonplace and include physical and mental illness and breakdown, stress and burn-out situations, depression and anxiety, as well as phenomena associated with physical and mental handicaps. In these situations correcting or adjusting techniques are used by many of us much of the time. In other words 'normal' or appropriate performance is caused by the deployment of appropriate stabilizers. Reliability of behaviour is caused by the overt and covert employment of correcting mechanisms. It is only when individuals do not have sufficient or adequate stabilizers to employ that they are regarded as handicapped or disturbed.

Let us take the example of an adult male who is behaviourally normal, and is required to enter hospital because of a physical abnormality requiring surgical intervention. An individual under such circumstances faces major stress, and is also placed in an environment that is strange in terms of its physical, social, and psychological structures. It is now a world where information is often in a strange language and requirements are new and unfamiliar. Under these circumstances the individual declines in self-image. This is partly due to internal and physical health reasons, but other aspects relate to the problems he confronts with the unfamiliar environment. The result is inhibition of his behaviour. His responses become slower so others repeat requests and gradually take over. He shows an inability to control the environment. Previously learned behaviours cannot be called upon as readily. He may forget names he knows well, be unable to express himself clearly, and will often indicate that he feels 'a fool' under such circumstances. He not only has a lack of knowledge to match the situation, he cannot draw on relevant knowledge to control the environment.

We have considerable knowledge about such processes. The work of Ley and Spelman (1965) demonstrated that people under physical stress situations retain less information, and are confused over it. There is some evidence that they are unable to 'hear' information effectively.

How can we reverse such behaviours? One way of doing so is to increase the environment in terms of familiar structures. In a hospital situation the environment is certainly structured, but it is not done in terms of the individual's own and familiar structures. Thus dissonance is set up and further breakdown results. The work of Prugh, already discussed, is particularly relevant. It is of interest that children with mother show much more dramatic and threatening behaviour for nursing staff which underlines the relevance of the model that we have suggested (i.e. responding with assertive behaviour which may be regarded as aggressive). Ferguson and Larsen (1987) note that a significant proportion of children who are hospitalized encounter psychological stress. These are often children entering hospital for surgical procedure. The authors suggest means of reducing such stress, including physical relaxation and guided imagery. This fits well with the concepts of familiarization and structure, while the kinaesthetic and visual components are very relevant to the regression model discussed later.

When familiar structures are present, and when familiarity increases, overt behaviour can be increased—although the observer may not always like the overt behaviour shown. This suggests ways in which we might control unwanted overt behaviour in other circumstances, namely by reducing the structure of the environment so that there is increased environmental unfamiliarity. The individual's self-image is decreased, which should to a large degree inhibit undesirable behaviour. The present authors have employed unfamiliarity effectively to inhibit destructive and hyperactive behaviours for short time periods. This phenomenon has been known for a long while, but no effective model in terms of understanding the dynamics has been put forward. Thus the practitioner rarely uses the knowledge to any advantage.

Behaviour and modalities

It is recognized in biology and psychology that behaviour tends to occur in a particular developmental sequence. Behaviour first develops within the tactile domain. In young infants this appears understandable in terms of the developing embryonic structures, for in the embryonic environment it is tactile responsiveness that is much to the fore. The visual modality is the next to develop, and later the processing of auditory information occurs. The development of modalities overlaps, but it appears that the later the onset of development of a modality, the greater its eventual command and interpretation of incoming stimuli. Young infants can modify linguistic output from a very early age but command of language occurs later than command of visual information. The importance of the sequencing of the three modalities from an evolutionary point of view is also noted. The developmental sequence of different areas is relevant, and even at the level of dendritic development, myelination and supporting tissue, there appears to be a sequence which is not inconsistent with the behavioural and rehabilitation model outlined here. For example, Dobbing (1975), Goldman (1975), and others suggest that there is a neural basis for hierarchical development of behaviour with development in certain areas of the brain preceding other areas. Restak (1979) notes that the visual cortex is established relatively early, but after the vestibular system, which plays a major role in co-ordination.

If certain types of systems develop before others, it may be reasonable to assume that the first stage acts as a foundation for the development of the next. In terms of modalities this creates a particular challenge, since it is apparent that loss of a modality such as vision requires the substitution of bridges from tactile to auditory. Fortunately, blindness from birth is comparatively rare amongst people with visual impairment. Many blind persons become more dependent on tactile imput than do unimpaired persons, and the more concrete aspects of audition, for example the recognition of 'sound shadows' due to the presence of building structures, can also be usefully employed by visually impaired persons in mobility training. Yet many visually impaired persons find it difficult, if not impossible, to learn braille, and persons who have recently become visually impaired often show major emotional stress and require long periods for adaptation. We would anticipate such behaviour from a consideration of the unfamiliarity-familiarity model. It is suggested that the behavioural model and its components might be employed to explain to visually impaired persons and their relatives, as well as staff working with them, the nature of this regression, its causes, together with concrete aids to help adapt to the stressful and unfamiliar situation. It is significant in this context that the self-image of visually impaired persons is known to be particularly poor, a phenomenon which can be modified to some degree with practical counselling and insight.

Many words used in our own language structure, and certainly the first words that are learned and used, relate to visual types of information. The development of an auditory language system is initially based on the presence of an effective visual language system, and this in turn is associated with the nature of tactile and kinaesthetic systems (Sokolov, 1969). Yet within the auditory modality the developmental nature of the system is even more apparent. Abstract words are defined, as a rule, by means of more concrete words. Thus gradually the language system becomes more and more remote from, and independent of, the visual system.

In terms of behaviour, the modalities also involve a certain range of control by an organism. A major differentiation between modalities appears to be the degree of proximity of origination of stimuli. Tactile and kinaesthetic systems relate to the immediate parts of the body and the impact of stimulation on or within that body. Such stimulation originates, in terms of impact and awareness, within the body of the young infant or on its surface. With visual information the source may originate at a considerable distance from the individual, while auditory information may be even more remote in origin and more diverse in source. Yet there are developmental controls over the range of accessibility to use of the modality. An example has been given in the auditory domain in terms of sequence of learning of words, but limitations can also be observed in the visual arena. For example, neonates first tend to focus at a distance of about 20 cm, suggesting the rest of the visual environment is a blur. It seems possible that such a phenomenon restricts visual impact of data, thus reducing the amount of irrelevant stimulation. Thus the amount of environmental input tends to be under developmental control. The senses represent building blocks by which a young infant gradually gains control first of its immediate environment, and later over a wide range of the external environment. This occurs through an interplay of mechanisms and sources of information. The individual gradually gains access to a wider range of information and increasing control of the environment.

Yet if there is a breakdown in incoming information, through some new type of task or information, it may be anticipated that the child will become particularly confused in those areas of information which have been most recently attained. Thus the individual is likely to show most disturbance in the tasks which are most recently learned. With increasing age the auditory modality is likely to become more and more prominent in this respect. There is a considerable amount of evidence to support such a model. It is apparent that people who suffer from confusional states and from traumatic accidents first lose recently learned material, and the regaining of material tends to be from earlier learned towards most recently learned information. Although there are many examples where the format outlined may not apply, for example in certain specific aphasias, it is apparent the model can act as a useful and preliminary guide.

Concrete and abstract language

Another dimension of behaviour, which we have not examined at this point, is the continuum of concrete to abstract learning, although it was discussed in relation to training continua. Concrete words are the first words to be used by young children, and they generally denote simple visual concepts. At a later age abstract qualities emerge, including words with complex meaning. It is generally agreed that around 12–13 years of age these abstract qualities come much to the fore (Piaget, 1952a).

In a variety of conditions which are characterized by behavioural disturbance, concrete words are employed where we would otherwise expect abstract processes to occur. There are a number of tests based on the concept of measuring concreteness of response, and this concreteness is used as a diagnostic sign within a variety of disease or mental health structures. Yet the point being made here is that a return to concrete language is a normal process designed to cope with the problems that confront an individual. For example, a young woman is given an auditory task which involves the use of abstract words, words which she does not always comprehend. Therefore she cannot undertake the task she is attempting. There are a number of routes she can follow. For example, she can ask individuals to define the words. If this is done it is likely that the person who defines the words for the individual does so in terms of previously learned concepts. There is nothing remarkable in this, for one can only envisage learning new information in terms of a combination of previously learned data which are familiar. The point is that, because of the nature of development, previous learning will normally be more concrete or visual, or more tactile and more gross, and less precise than the concepts which are now being learned.

Gross to specific behaviour

In order to understand the procedure further it is important to recognize another dimension of behaviour. Behaviour normally proceeds from the gross to the specific. Once specific learning has taken place it is likely to be internalized or become covert. Young infants show gross behaviour as they attempt new tasks. Their behaviour is massive and involves a wide range of gross muscle involvement. Gradually, as the youngster gains command of performance, so the behaviour becomes more specific and what is now redundant movement and action disappears. The same type of process is seen in much later learning, even though there is transfer from previous learned skills. For example, an individual who learns to ski for the first time in adult life will show gross motor behaviour and in-coordination. Gradually he will gain control of his skis with redundant behaviour dropping out, resulting in a smooth performance and much less expenditure of energy. The introduction of newness in any form will lead to the reassertion of gross behaviour to some degree, even though the individual has previously learned the basic task. Learning to drive a new car will promote gross and redundant behaviour, as well as inappropriate behaviour. Behaviour becomes refined as the individual practises. The same behaviour is seen in learning tasks with a high level of transfer involved. For example, one of us is learning to play the organ. Even after many years of piano playing, experienced finger movements become more gross and muscle cramps result from simple organ exercises. A further example involves a project on which we are working. Arab students with first degrees are involved in a Canadian International Development Agency project. As part of their work they have been required to write material in English. Their motor skills in Arabic are immaculate, but without exception, requirements to write in a foreign language from right to left initially produced writing which was similar to English-speaking children 6−8 years of age. This is a particularly pertinent example because it suggests that where over-learning of a specific skill has taken place, the learning of a closely allied but different skill, results in specific and general problems in additional skill areas.

The point of such examples is that much of the behaviour shown by individuals undergoing rehabilitation is not an unusual phenomenon associated only with disabled persons, but a process required by all of us embarking on new learning. The general nature of rehabilitation, when recognized, will do much to affect our perception of recovery and relearning. The behavioural examples also serve to note that disability in the eyes of society is a phenomenon of traditional classification. With growth of technology, and therefore technical skill, and the requirements of social integration across foreign communities, the catalogue of disabilities will inevitably rise. It may be wise to reconsider whether disability is a suitable label.

Overt to covert behaviour

However, behaviour does not just conform to a gross to specific movement; it also involves a process of internalization and automatization (Sternberg, 1985). In most instances the learning of language is an external process involving a range of gross behaviour, and in some instances inappropriate behaviour. A few children seem to accumulate language knowledge without much speech, and speak almost from the start in short sentences. However this may relate to the size of steps that specific individuals can absorb during learning. Eventually the language becomes specific, and in problem-solving situations it reduces in terms of its volume until it may, when it is not actually necessary for the conveying of information to other persons, become internalized. Some minor motor movement may still occur in the laryngeal area and can be recorded from electrode contact, but the speech appears to have been internalized. But Sokolov (1969) has noted that speech motor tension increases when an abstract problem-solving task is introduced. Thus, although there appears to be a continuum of development from overt to covert, the process may be reversed with introduction of new and difficult tasks. This also appears, according to Sokolov, to be related to how people access their memory for words. Speech motor tension is greatest in people with a tendency for motor memory for words, somewhat less intense for those with an auditory memory, and less still in those whose access is visual memory. If the abstract task is reformulated in visual terms (i.e. an outline scheme or model) the amount of speech motor tension decreases. Both increased education and age appear to be associated with a reduction in speech motor tension.

A model of behavioural rehabilitation

It may now be helpful to put this information into a comprehensive, if tentative, model. Figure 9 outlines the impact of a new task on performance. The figure shows the development of three modalities over time: tactile followed by visual and then auditory. Although the diagram shows the auditory modality to be the most developed, this is not to suggest that visual and tactile learning ceases, but rather, in the reasonably mature individual, it is likely that much learning takes place within the auditory modality, the other modalities having been established earlier.

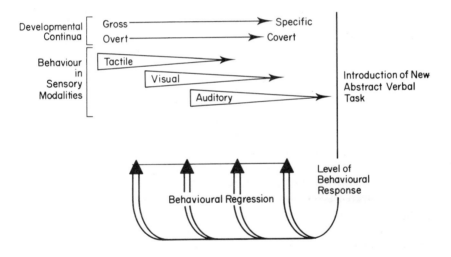

Figure 9. An example of suggested impact of a new task on performance.

When a new task or new stress is introduced to a normal individual, we may expect a variety of phenomena to occur. First of all, within any specific modality, behaviour may be expected to cycle to a more primitive level of performance. Covert or internalized language may be expected to become overt. Under extreme conditions it may also become incoherent, because the stress has broken the smooth sequence of internalized language structure. At this level it may be assumed that a large amount of redundancy is involved in the language process, which perhaps has some relevance to the incoherent and disturbed type of speech found in a number of abnormal conditions. Overt language at first will be coherent and may involve elaborated code, but under stress will become more restricted, perhaps paralleling the socialinguistic levels of language described by Bernstein (1967). The restricted code has been identified as a possible hindrance to children's school progress (Edwards and Giles, 1984). The emotional content of the language may also rise. Thus there is a trend from complex, abstract and logical language to concrete, simple and emotional language.

There is also a regression in other areas of behaviour. The individual may show sufficient breakdown that he regresses from auditory to visual, and under extreme stress, tactile response patterns. Visual or tactile may come to dominate in the performance. Thus an individual confronted with a new task in the auditory modality may regress to a visual level of performance, and an individual confronted with a visual task may regress to a tactile level of performance. There is no reason why, under extreme forms of stress, regression from auditory through visual to tactile performance should not occur. However the argument here is not that this regressive behaviour is some type of abnormal breakdown of the individual, but is, in the first instance, a psychologically normal and effective process by which the individual attempts to attain or regain control of his environment, and deal with the new situation confronting him by restructuring response patterns at a more simple level. Thus regression is used here not to denote abnormality of behaviour, but rather to describe a normal process which may assist the individual to continue with a coherent performance.

We now have a model which helps to explain why certain behaviour occurs. But more than this it provides us with a means of indicating what behaviour is likely to occur under specific conditions. It should also tell us the types of learning and emotional structures that are needed in planning rehabilitation programmes. As indicated earlier, such a model should apply across diagnostic categories. The degree of complexity of behaviour and the level at which the individual is functioning determine the point on the model where the rehabilitation programme is commenced. Application of the model may be complicated by anomalies. For example, a visually impaired person may not have the visual modality available to him. Since this represents one of the major building blocks within the developmental sequence described, substitutes become very necessary. Yet even in cases of hearing loss (e.g. deaf mutism or aphasia) the teaching of a sign language or finger spelling is still associated with tongue and lip movements. Work reported by Sokolov (1969) indicates speech motor tension in both of these conditions.

In the system described above baseline assessment becomes a critical requirement in order to design and develop the remedial process. The type of assessment that needs to take place must differ dramatically from the type of diagnostic analysis that has traditionally formed the basis of psychological assessment. By definition the learning carried out must relate to the performance that we wish to encourage. Such a process involves the availability of curriculum, a sequence of tasks, a transfer or generalization programme, adequate apparatus and knowledgeable staff set within a client-oriented system. It also assumes appropriate environments in which to carry out rehabilitation.

Variability and cyclic behaviour

We might ask why individuals show high or low aggression, or why they show wide ranges of variation in their level of responsiveness. It is suggested that the rate of responsiveness is affected not only by general levels of motivation, but by factors such as familiarity of the task, the physical environment, and the people within the person's environment. The difficulty level of the tasks and the challenges confronting the individual are relevant in this context.

There are other factors which are extremely important in determining the level of responsiveness and therefore learning. But the responses show what has been described earlier as cyclic behaviour. If we are able to predict the changes in familiarity of the environment, if we are able to describe the stress of a particular environment, and the learning ability of the individual concerned, then we may get some idea of how effective the individual is going to be at any particular point in time. Unfortunately environments, situations, tasks and activity level of individuals vary constantly throughout the day, and therefore rapid and considerable changes may be expected in the individual's performance from point to point within the day.

Probably most of us employ a variety of mechanisms to counteract these various stresses and changes. When we have learned effectively, despite changes in the situation, we produce a remarkably consistent level of performance. Even so, normal individuals may show great variation under certain conditions. For example, long periods of driving a car can result in an increase in error rate, hunger can result in high irritability levels, and illness or extreme unfamiliarity or stress produces a change in response rate and accuracy. We would expect these phenomena to be much worse for handicapped individuals.

One of the marked characteristics of handicapped individuals, reported in the literature by Gunzburg (1968) and many others, is the high variability of performance. Mentally handicapped people, for example, are not just remarkable because of their low level of performance, but because they show enormous variability in their behaviour. This variability is also true of many persons recovering from brain injury and those suffering from mental illness. It is also true of many criminals.

Oscillation of behaviour

As seen elsewhere, new learning is particularly vulnerable to intrusions of stress and unfamiliarity. There is very considerable evidence that traumatic events damage new learning before they harm earlier learning. We therefore may suppose that around recent learning there is a period for establishment or permanency, and during this period the behaviour may be easily disrupted by fairly minor stresses within the environment (see Figure 10). We refer to this as oscillation in behaviour, because it seems to come and go depending on the circumstances. Because of the nature and sequencing of learning we would expect, in normal persons, that auditory and linguistic behaviours would be most vulnerable to oscillation effects because they represent the bulk of new learning. Cycling would be expected to be much less apparent in visual learning, and with tactile learning even less still. This is illustrated in the figure on oscillation and performance.

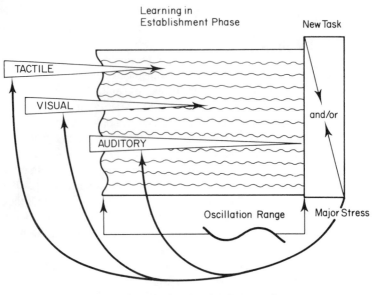

Learning in
Establishment Phase

New Task

TACTILE

VISUAL

and/or

AUDITORY

Oscillation Range

Major Stress

Alternative levels of regression

Figure 10. Oscillation and performance in individual behaviour.

Because handicapped people are slower at learning it could be suggested that their more recent learning remains in a more vulnerable condition for a rather lengthier period of time than non-handicapped individuals, thus accounting for the very wide range in variability of performance which is found in most handicapped persons. Further, it would be expected that individuals who are elderly, or individuals who are suffering from mental illnesses, would be even more vulnerable at particular times of the day because of interaction with other normal but stressful processes. For example hunger and fatigue, and thoughts of disease and deterioration, would further lower such individuals' thresholds and thus they might be expected to show greater oscillation during these times. But the situation may be more extreme than this. These examples suggest that it is not just new learning that is vulnerable, but also other behaviours. When such individuals come against major stress then it might be anticipated that behaviour would regress beyond the area referred to as normal oscillation. When the stress is removed recovery would be expected; thus a wide oscillation effect may be produced. This degree of oscillation is, we suggest, what is classically recognized as abnormality of behaviour in individuals suffering from mental health problems.

Environment—structure and stability

With this background in mind it becomes appropriate to discuss the nature of structuring of environment, because when training is commenced it should normally be at the concrete level. Physical constructs and surroundings are needed in which to provide the training process.

There is a continuum from highly concrete activities to activities which might be regarded as more abstract. The concrete activities illustrate the phenomenon of structure to a very large degree. Tasks must take place at a particular place, at a particular time, in a particular manner. Simple vocational tasks fit this bill very well, as do a variety of motor tasks. Individuals do not often have to move far from base, and generally have somebody who monitors behaviour or informs them of the necessary steps to take. There is no long-term temporal sequence to the behaviour or to the learning, for once the learning has been carried out, the activity is repeated in much the same way at all times, at all stages. This is one reason why vocational types of activities are relatively easy to teach, and why a wide range of very severely handicapped people appear to learn them extremely readily. It may also be why vocational rehabilitation is, on its own, severely limiting, and does not transfer to other settings.

Much residential behaviour falls into the same pattern, and institutions are an extreme form of this. They are precisely organized and controlled. Generally the learning required is basic and specific. However, as rehabilitation workers quickly recognized, as they placed vocationally competent people into the workforce, other skills were necessary in order to enable the individual to survive in the community. By and large vocational and residential training at their most basic are more concrete than either social or leisure time education skills. And certainly the skills in the more advanced stages of the latter are seen as much more abstract than the former. This is apparently because the nature of abstract learning is associated with a breakdown in external structure; for example, making social choices when moving into the community, or making decisions while shopping or catching buses. All these involve behaviour which is generally unmonitored and often shows diversity of stimulation, resulting in immediate decisions which have to be applied effectively to the situation.

What we see occurring is a process from structured to unstructured training in which temporal readiness and stability of the task changes dramatically. Under these circumstances the most obvious way to ensure that an individual performs adequately is to:

1). make the structures as concrete as possible in the first instance, and
2). recognize the structure has to be internalized in order for the individual to apply it when he is on his own without the usual external constructs which maintain or contain his behaviour.

For the traumatized or elderly person, previously learned material which is forgotten or not readily accessed may be tantamount to a new learning situation. Under such circumstances it is therefore expected from the model that these individuals will also regress. The behaviour of such persons is often seen as depression, whereas in our model, although the behaviour will demonstrate aspects of depression, it is more reasonable to regard it as anxiety and stress reaction behaviour in an individual who can no longer attain the necessary baseline for performance in a particular situation. This is exemplified in the writings of Fry (1986) on stress and depression in elderly persons. The obvious behavioural recourse is to reduce the demands in the particular situation and provide the environmental crutches which will enable the person to stabilize and then develop from the new behavioural baseline which occurs. Obviously if a person is rapidly deteriorating (elderly persons) this may not be very easy to do. A person may have stabilized, but may still be required to function in a situation beyond his or her capability at that point in time. A sensitivity towards impact of environment, and a need to constantly restructure environment, seems highly desirable, and should be recognized by personnel and by other individuals living closely with the person.

The idea of structuring the environment is not a new concept, and has been referred to by a variety of people in different circumstances (e.g. in controlling wandering behaviour in elderly persons Hussion, 1981; restructuring the environment in modifying children's aberrant behaviour, Tymchuk, 1974). Earlier papers, particularly in the field of mental handicap, spoke of structuring of environments but rarely described what was meant by such phrases. More recent work by Brown and Hughson (1980) has attempted to define what is meant by structure. Other workers such as Whelan and Speake (1984) and Gold (1973) have given clear examples of what this means in the field of training handicapped adults. Basically it implies who does the training, where the training is done, when it is done and what is done. The examples here only relate to specific training samples. We require a generalizable model which will involve structuring in environmental settings, whether or not the learning environment is regarded as training, school education or socialization within the family setting. The model discussed earlier provides an example in terms of the constructs which should be employed. If learning goes from concrete to abstract, then environments themselves must go from concrete to abstract. If the learning situation goes from tactile to visual to auditory, then the type of stimulation applied by the environment must go through these three modalities at the same rate, or behaviour becomes fixated at a particular level. A normal individual, who has high self-esteem and is seeking stimulation, will naturally proceed through the tactile, visual and auditory modalities, but this book is about people who do not proceed through these three modalities effectively. Therefore additional aids and supports are required in order to ensure that the environment provides the right type of stimulation at the right time through the right type of person.

Internal and external structure

The importance of development of self-image has been noted, and it is suggested that it is correlated with a process of internalizing knowledge, structure and processes from the external environment. It has been argued that self-image is boosted by greater control of one's environment, but that this control cannot occur until the individual has learned certain aspects and principles of cognitive structure. Learning is at first often at a conscious level and is slow and clumsy. Gradually, as the individual becomes more effective, these structures become internalized and to a large degree unconscious or as Sternberg states, automatic. If one accepts Sternberg's (1985) arguments about intelligence, then we must perceive this internalization of structure as a growth in cognitive power, thus self-image is linked to the development of intelligence.

Individuals need, during early development, to receive structured control, including direction by adults, or the structure of more experienced and knowledgeable persons. This is observed in parenting models and within school systems. These structures relax as individuals grow and develop.

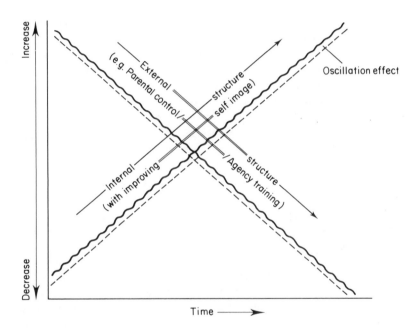

Figure 11. Schematic representation of external support during development and gradual improvement in self-image and internal structure.

Figure 11 shows a schematic representation of how these processes may be linked. With reduced external structure and control there should be an increase in internalized knowledge and the positive development of self-image. Even if this system is accepted, and its relevance to rehabilitation noted, one is struck by the fact that in society and within all dimensions of rehabilitation it is assumed that these changes are linear and that one process automatically leads to another. Thus the types of structures that are found in school systems at more advanced levels, or available within our adult community, assume that individuals have internalized structure and therefore can have greater freedom and choice.

But it is apparent that individuals develop at different rates, and nowhere is this more true than in the various dimensions of social health, where mental breakdown, premature ageing, deterioration and disability interfere with the normal or regular growth systems. Further, it has been suggested that oscillation or cycles of behaviour are very common, and no more so than when one is dealing with individuals who are undertaking new learning, for such new learning, once just established, is much more vulnerable to stress than more established learning.

It is at these front-line levels that we see regression and progression interacting. Instead of a linear relationship which can easily be plotted, there would appear to be both rises and falls in behavioural efficiency. There will be falls in self-image and externalization of internal behaviour structure as automatic and reciprocating mechanisms in individuals come into play in association with problems in learning new material. There must be a recognition of such processes by parents and agencies, and effective procedures must be built to take them into account. Similar behavioural regression is found in normal learning, and simple directions to change the level of performance can make learning more efficient. For example, in teaching any court sport such as squash, a new learner may advance from a simple to a more complex service. Behaviour during the mastery of the new serve may disintegrate through a breakdown in co-ordination. An instruction to go back to a previous service for a few moments and then return to the new situation can result in a regaining of behavioural control. This form of interplay between instructor and instructed, and the recognition of behavioural regression effects, is very important in rehabilitation.

Individuals do not need to work nor perform permanently under the structured portion of the model. They need to be encouraged to advance their behaviour as they adapt. It is important that our social structures specifically provide for some acceleration, by gradually minimizing external structure, and provoking greater reliance on the individual as a stimulus to further development.

It is only necessary, during regression, to increase structural support systems to a baseline where the individual can perform accurately, and then provide the necessary stimulation to bring him or her back to a more advanced level of behaviour as illustrated in the above example. This oscillation, it is suggested, occurs to all of us, whether it is during a learning session or on a diurnal basis as we become more fatigued or more restless, or over longer cycles due to stress, frustration or minor physical illness. Further, it results from more pervasive factors such as depression or more long-lasting impacts such as organic damage. Yet even in the latter cases one must be aware that growth and change can be stimulated by the application of the types of structures outlined, because recovery in the brain is at least partly a reaction to the stimulation that is provided to the individual.

In many instances of major stress, sudden drops in performance are likely, and they indicate a need for rapid increase in external structure and control. Improvement in individuals, in terms of self-image and internalized structure, may be of a more gradual nature, suggesting that external control systems to induce and support recovery should be reduced gradually. This underlines the importance of flexibility in teaching style, and the relevance of a thorough knowledge of principles guiding or causing behavioural change.

CHAPTER FIVE

Assessment in rehabilitation

Introduction

The aim of this chapter is to present an overview of the processes and procedures of assessment in what has been broadly defined as rehabilitation education (Brown, 1984b). A considerable amount of effort has been put into the assessment of disabled persons over the past 25 years. Many of the ideas which are expressed here have been gradually taking form in various clinics, and research and demonstration centres. Using the model described earlier, an attempt is made to put together a rationale for assessment, and to integrate these ideas as a basis for future practice.

Review of assessment

In order to consider the issue of assessment in educational and rehabilitation processes it is necessary to review briefly four of its major functions. As indicated by Clarke and Clarke (1976), assessment is necessary to describe an individual at a particular point in time, in terms of intellectual, social, emotional, educational and allied variables, with reference to a normative or contrast population. Secondly, the function of assessment is to predict performance of an individual at a future point in time. Thirdly, assessment provides a profile of assets and deficits in order to determine a starting point for further intervention or training. Fourthly, assessment provides an objective means of monitoring progress of an individual, or a group of individuals, over time. This last category leads to further implications for assessment in the programme evaluation aspects of service delivery.

Many traditional forms of assessment, such as psychometric testing, were directed to what might be called native ability or capacity, and were concerned with inherent abilities that are usually only inferred from standard test items in a mix of genetic and environmental interaction (Hebb, 1949). Over the years an anti-psychometric movement has grown up, particularly in rehabilitation and special education. Many people have asked questions about the significance of scores on psychometric tests and an individual's ability to adapt or survive in the natural community. Furthermore, questions about the extent to which reported scores on specific tests are considered to be stable within an individual, and the relevance these results have for the prediction of future performance or success in the community, have been raised. The matter of predictive ability of tests within the field of disability, and particularly mental handicap, has been discussed at length by writers such as Cobb (1966). In summary, his work suggests that long-term prediction is currently ineffective, and where short-term prediction is examined it seems to be most effective in some social and in certain motor skill areas. The work of people such as Grant (1971) suggests that prediction by supervisors of the likely success of disabled persons in work tasks is very poor, and considerably underestimates actual success on these tasks. Test results should not be used for long-term prediction, and when used for short-term prediction they should be employed for specific prescriptive purposes.

As has already been stated, another purpose of assessment is in the area of describing, categorizing or labelling an individual at a particular point in time, but with a movement away from standard psychometric testing, much criticism has been levelled at such labelling processes. The practice of diagnosing areas of behavioural disability through conventional testing has little relevance to the ability to provide prescriptive and powerful teaching interventions directed to improvement in performance.

Many government services and allied service systems have conventionally attached financial costs to programmes and provided funds on a *per diem* basis, the amount being determined by the label attached to the individual. In evaluating the role of assessment it is important to separate reasons of financial expediency or administrative convenience from the legitimate requirements of remediation, intervention and treatment.

Although it is recognized that many authorities may wish to use assessment techniques for the purpose of classification, there is little evidence to support such a process. It is also argued, from the point of view of the model presented, that the generic nature of behaviour, underlying different disabling conditions, argues against any formal sense of classification. Furthermore, the degree of variability in performance from one occasion to another makes it unlikely that any classification based on any particular record or records of an individual would have any long-term justification.

Many behavioural practitioners, recognizing the inadequacies of conventional psychometric instruments, have attempted to look at alternatives (e.g. Feuerstein, 1979; Haywood, 1984). There has been an attempt to devise new instruments or modify existing ones to try to tap into the dynamic learning potential of individual clients. An interest is being shown in the process of learning rather than simply the level of performance.

The major shift in assessment has been in the area of functionality. Behaviourists in the field of education and rehabilitation (Halpern and Fuhrer, 1984) have reviewed some of the major work in this area. These researchers have delineated the difference between impairment, disability and handicap, and thus developed a matrix of needs in assessment as determined by the domain that is being measured. In the functional approach to assessment, both summative and formative measures are used. The formative measures of assessment are detailed with specific observations of task-specific behaviour, including measurement of individual items of behaviour that are necessary to the larger and complex skill areas.

Primary and secondary handicaps

The development of assessment procedures and their relationship to the model also raises the concept of primary and secondary handicaps. The recognition that there is no one cause of a particular individual's functioning, though there may be a precipitating cause or causes, underlines an important concept. A transdisciplinary assessment process is required, and it assumes that the accumulation of environmental effects and deficits may make life much more difficult for any individual and may handicap that individual much further. The concept of impairment, disability and handicap, as described by Halpern and Fuhrer (1984), speaks to this type of process. However, in terms of the rehabilitation model described, we believe it is important to examine and record the nature of primary and secondary handicaps. One of the areas of programme development and change to be addressed involves the secondary as well as primary handicaps that exist in an individual's lifestyle.

Primary negative impact

This refers to the initial, or precipitating, condition which causes the first handicap to the individual. It may be the major handicap, but not necessarily. For example, an abnormal genetic condition in a young child can be regarded as the primary negative impact, and may result to some degree in retarded intelligence. The condition may also result in facial features which are distorted. This latter problem may precipitate, along with the mild loss of intelligence, negative responses from the environment such as withdrawal from the individual, and rejection by parents. These effects may have far more impact on the individual's development than the original condition.

The primary negative impact may be genetic or environmental. In the field of mental handicap it is quite frequently an adverse environment, though there are individuals such as Jensen (1970) who have argued that polygenetic inheritance may also be responsible. Outside the field of mental handicap, in the area of physical trauma, such as brain injury from a car accident, obviously the primary impact is an environmental one. In the field of severe retardation it is frequently inherited.

Secondary negative impact

This refers to conditions which impinge on the individual generally because of the presence of a primary negative impact. Examples of this have been given above. Secondary negative impact can include such situations as sending a child by bus to a special school. It is known that children who travel for one or two hours a day can become extremely fatigued by such a process. Therefore their learning is handicapped by the travelling itself. In this case secondary impact is added to primary impact. Secondary negative impacts are often multiple factors that do not occur in isolation. Furthermore, the individual concerned with behavioural processes is frequently in a position to modify much of the secondary impact. It should be noted that the secondary impact may, individually or cumulatively, have much more adverse effect on the individual than the primary condition. Table 1 illustrates some examples of primary and secondary negative impact and it is recommended that those working in the field should always list in case files and reports the past and current primary and secondary impacts which have had a negative or adverse effect on the child or adult.

Table 1. Examples of primary and secondary causation in impairment.

Primary	Secondary
Genetic defect	Long distance of travel to school
Brain injury	Inadequate play material
Adverse environment	Negative attitudes from and between parents
Sensory impairment	Poor nutrition
Disease	Inadequate verbal models
	Inconsistent learning environment
	Inappropriate clothing
	Experiences contributing to poor self-image and poor motivation
	Residential relocations (particularly for the elderly person)
	New work settings

Primary causes may be relegated to secondary impact.
Secondary causation may sometimes be elevated to primary causation.
Accumulated secondary causations may have more damaging effect than primary causation.

If one wishes to consider the importance of impact on an individual in a broader manner, the positive impacts should also be recognized. Primary positive impacts may account for why some individuals are particularly effective. This may relate to good genetic endowment or very positive environmental circumstances or to a combination of these factors. In rehabilitation it is essential to know the nature of positive or potentially positive secondary impact on an individual for such conditions, if they are available, or if they can be provided, for may dramatically change the learning situation and therefore the performance of an individual. Social workers and psychologists often note a secondary positive impact in terms of a supportive family, but it is suggested that it is necessary to go one stage further, and capitalize on such situations to the greatest advantage of the individual concerned.

It is apparent from what is said above that secondary and sometimes primary positive factors are associated with the environment. It is important to recognize that we are talking not just about social, psychological or educational aspects of the environment, but physical circumstances as well, such as the design of a home or accessibility to the urban or rural community in which an individual lives.

Variability in growth

Variability in growth and performance is also a consideration in assessment and programming. Figure 12 illustrates some material based on the work of Gunzburg

(1968). It indicates the times at which skills were gained by individuals who were normal, and individuals who were labelled severely retarded. The latter group functioned below an IQ of 55. The importance of these data is not only that they show the expected delayed development of handicapped youngsters, but also that they indicate a few of the children who were handicapped learned as rapidly as a few of the children who were said to be of average intelligence. This is interesting in its own right. Of course the considerable period over which children gained such skills shows that learning occurred over a wide age range. Perhaps it is of greater significance that the variability of learning amongst the severely handicapped group was of considerable magnitude. It took about 9 years for 75 per cent of them to learn the particular skill, whereas it took only 3 years for 75 per cent of the normal group to obtain such skills. This suggests that variability amongst the handicapped persons as described in Gunzburg's study is about three times that of normal children.

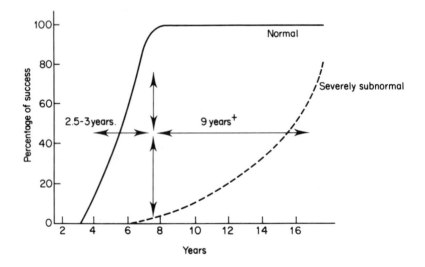

Figure 12. Ability to play simple table games (eg. dominoes). (*Adapted, with permission, from Gunzburg, H.C.*, Social Competence and Mental Handicap, *Baillière Tindall and Cassell, 1968.*.

Variable growth rate, as interpreted here in the broad context of learning skills, appears important. Firstly it shows that individuals change and go on growing over a very long period of time, even though they are quite severely handicapped. Secondly, and more importantly, it shows that individuals who have the same broad cognitive label learn skills at very different times. Such variability obviously argues for individualized instruction, but it also points to the fact that instructors must recognize the enormous range of variability which occurs.

It is amongst handicapped persons that individual approaches to assessment and learning are needed. Unless each person can be provided with a specific kind of education, it is unlikely that they will progress effectively. It is also apparent, if there is this wide range of variability amongst people showing a narrow band of intelligence, that tests such as the IQ will be unable to predict the likelihood of improved performance. Uniqueness appears to be the rule of the day, and therefore efforts to produce tests of a more normative variety, and to use them to provide data to explain human behaviour amongst disabled persons, are unlikely to give us any great insights into the nature of human variability. We may categorize behaviour, we may be able to classify it, we may even be able to describe it en masse, yet the processes that go on in the development of behaviour are likely, through over-use of these procedures, to be ignored.

Normative and criterion-referenced testing

Much of the preceding material is based on concepts associated with normative assessment. That is, instances where individuals, when assessed, are compared with a range of other individuals which represent a normal sample of the population or a particular sample from a specified population. Such standardized measures are still frequently employed, and have their uses for resolving particular problems. For example, where an individual may appear to be under-functioning badly in specific areas, a standardized cognitive test may indicate average or above-average ability. Such test materials are often based on a wide sample of behaviours, and therefore give little specific or precise information which can be employed for zeroing in on baseline needs and programme requirements for the individual. Such measures, as indicated earlier, have little predictive function and therefore even if the test data are used for classification, they are unlikely to indicate how the individual will progress in future years.

In many areas, and specifically in relation to the development of programme material, criterion reference testing has developed (Baine, 1978). Tests devised in this way give little information for comparison with normative populations, but they do indicate whether an individual can or cannot carry out a specific task. In the field of disability this is probably the most essential requirement. For example, if an individual can carry out certain social skills or certain mechanical skills effectively it is not of very great interest whether he is of average ability or of low average ability. The criterion is whether or not he can carry out the task. Such test structures have been very important in terms of the development of programmed material and subsequently the development and application of what has become to be called the individual programme plan. Effective programming planning, which is devised for specific individuals, can be associated with criterion-referenced testing. By these means plans can be put forward with very specific goals, and with very specific criteria to indicate whether the individual has attained or not attained these goals. The role of criterion-referenced testing, as a psychometric measure, is extremely important and should be employed very much more, not only by psychologists but by teachers and rehabilitation educators who wish to devise precise programme planning for individual children or adults.

A developmental approach to assessment

At the summative level a wide range of behavioural checklists have been developed with a view to the identification of functioning in social and emotional areas, daily living skills, recreation and leisure, home living and vocational areas. The approach attempts to emphasize the developmental model as opposed to a deficit model, and is concerned with adaptive behaviour in natural settings. The growth of this area of assessment has also led to other measures that are not primarily directed to the individual, but are concerned with environmental and ecological variables impinging on the individual and affecting his or her functioning. The association or interactions between the individual and the environment becomes a critical matter.

More recently research and assessment techniques have been concerned with looking at the process of learning, including the cognitive processes, which involve the strategies that people employ to solve problems, carry out activities, or perform skills. Much more work will be needed in this area, for it holds out more hope in terms of prediction and for the development of prescriptive treatment and training opportunities.

The concept of modifiability of intelligence which has grown in recent years (Feuerstein, 1979) suggests that intervention of one kind or another may affect the outcome of behaviour within a particular individual. As indicated in our model, such changes may occur through natural processes, or possibly through intervention processes. Such a belief system argues against the simple classification of individuals using the results of any type of assessment on any one occasion.

Regardless of the results from a specific assessment, intervention, whether natural or designed by rehabilitation workers, may influence the subsequent direction the individual takes in terms of skill development. Thus it is unlikely that the assessment results on one occasion will necessarily predict what an individual will accomplish, though trends may be established over long time periods. This last statement suggests that assessment at one point in time cannot be used alone as a determinant of development, because what has happened prior to assessment will also be part of the general structure which determines, along with future events, the path that the individual travels. The multidimensional aspects of human functioning, associated with events over time, are extremely complex. The argument is not that it is impossible to predict, but that at this stage of development there are insufficient measures at sufficiently varied points in time to carry out prediction effectively.

Assessment information is of little use unless it can be interpreted. Interpretation is dependent in part on the understanding that practitioners may have of the body of knowledge in rehabilitation, their perceptions of human behaviour, and the events in the natural environment. Descriptors of individual performance or behaviours are, on their own, very limited. Interpretation of assessment information within an environment is an important issue in the model proposed in this book. The model is dependent upon the systematic organization of assessment information with its application to intervention techniques.

Baseline behaviour, on any one particular occasion, is also subject to error. The further the scores on any particular occasion deviate from the mean or average scores of a population, the more likely are retest results to be higher than on the first occasion. This phenomenon, known as regression to the mean, is one that should be taken into account by those who undertake intervention processes (Clarke, Clarke and Brown, 1956). Because of this, and the difficulties inherent in measuring error effects precisely, it is essential, particularly when assessing the effects of intervention strategies, to attempt to minimize error in terms of baseline assessment. For this reason it is recommended, when providing baselines, prior to intervention of any particular performance, that at least two initial scores should be obtained. This is consistent with Cuvo's (1979) recommendations. In this fashion the tester can get some measure of the variability of performance. If the tester wishes to ensure that results are interpreted cautiously, then the higher of the two scores should be taken as an indication of baseline prior to intervention stategy occurring. Alternatively, an average of the two scores may be taken. Wide variability would, of course, argue for some further assessment prior to undertaking the intervention strategy, a phenomenon which is common in disabled individuals. Such a technique is not ideal, and error still remains. However, it is one way of overcoming a major difficulty when dealing with individuals who are likely to have very low scores on initial assessment and are almost bound to rise on second testing, regardless of whether intervention is employed or not. The use of double baselines rarely occurs in the development or assessment of programme strategies, and further, the importance of such measures in providing a more reliable baseline for indicating later progress to parents or clients seems to us ethical and professionally responsible.

Rating scales are notoriously unreliable under certain conditions, and also give rise to assessment errors. For example, if staff are not well trained in administering the scales, then it is likely that the results will not represent the best estimates of the individual's performance. Furthermore, it is obvious that different staff measuring the individual on the same occasion independently may provide different results. Some argue that in such cases highly skilled staff should be employed in the use of rating scales. We do not believe that this is necessary in many cases, but it is important that the staff, or the observers involved, for they may be parents or other people having close contact with the individual, do receive some training in the administration of such tests. The Adaptive Functioning Index (Marlett, 1971), for example, can, once staff are trained to administer the scales, show very high reliability in the order of 0.8 or 0.9, but without such training the results may be much lower, 0.2 or 0.3, which is useless in terms of providing a baseline or a description of the individuals. Even if staff are trained through workshops which may be of very short duration, high reliability levels may drop after a fairly brief period of time. In a recent quality-of-life study it was found necessary to ensure that staff were updated each year in terms of their rating skills, for without this reliability would drop considerably (Brown, Bayer and MacFarlane, 1986). It is therefore necessary not only to provide brief workshops where staff learn to rate individuals independently, but where there are differences, to encourage discussion between each pair of raters so that there is a resolution to the problems. This means establishing clear criteria in terms of what specifically is being measured and what specific words actually mean. For example, the rating statement 'Is able to use local transit skills' may mean very different skills in different environments or may represent different skills to different people. Once these differences are ironed out it is still, nevertheless, necessary periodically to provide revision for the staff.

There are several other considerations with regard to the interpretation of assessment that should be highlighted. In the context of functional assessments it is not uncommon to see behaviours identified with no conclusions made in terms of relationship of these items of behavioural data to overall functioning. Within the field this has been identified as the baseline on which one builds further programmatic events. Again the assumption is that the rehabilitation practitioner will be able to identify the next stage of training or level of intervention, provided there is some systematic set of stages or phases by which people learn skills. Although there is some research evidence which indicates that prerequisite skills may be required before moving on to other aspects of learning, such evidence has only been documented for certain specialized skill areas. It is known that many aspects of psychological and social behaviour may have certain prior learning sequences for their acquisition. Therefore baselines of these achievements are important for determining what is necessary for the next training sequence. It is at this stage that the trainer requires sophistication for determining how to apply the theoretical constructs from the model in a useful way to help the individual who needs to learn specific clusters of behaviour. It is suggested that the model can lead to a more systematic or structured development of assessment techniques that could measure environment and its interactions with disabled individuals.

Assessment provides for baseline, and for monitoring of performance during the administration of a task with a view to feeding the results into the process of further goal-setting and task selection, including modification of the existing task when it has not been learned effectively. This concept of assessment, which is clearly outlined by Whelan and Speake (1984), requires the specification of specific goals and particular teaching procedures along with criteria for success. Such specifications are made in advance of programme application and should result from the development of IPPs. Unfortunately the criteria for success, which often relate quite artificially to the arbitrary selection of a specific number of accurately performed trials, may bear no relation to whether the individual is able to utilize the skill learned, or whether the behaviour can be integrated into subsequent situations on a long-term basis. This has implications for both over-learning and transfer. It is an issue addressed in the model described, in that the model represents a continuous developmental process rather than a series of isolated tasks.

As indicated earlier, some writers (e.g. Baine, 1978) have advocated criterion-referenced testing, but the issue raised above is not taken into account. Such a process is possible provided one sets up the necessary training and testing sequences. Yet the process of criterion-referenced assessment is a major step forward, and elements of the process are invaluable for the design and development of future curriculum packages.

Assessment and individual programme planning

The individual programme plan, or individual education plan, which came into effect in the United States as a result of Public Law 94-142 and relates to education for all children, has within its design, opportunities for future planning and the development of skills and opportunities for children. It also underlines the need for multidisciplinary assessment which, in turn, necessitates the involvement of a wide range of personnel and interested others, such as parents, working with the child. In programme planning meetings specific goals are set and are communicated to all parties concerned. Procedures to be employed and timelines are incorporated. This, again, fits well with the model put forward, though it is suggested that the model itself provides additional components which would be valuable within the IPP approach. It is also relevant in terms of the development of individual programme plans which provide for the setting of goals in a wide range of areas, recognizing the transdisciplinary nature of the programmes that are developed. Unfortunately, as Marlett (1986) indicates, very often these new models of programme planning are formalized into rigid administrative structures on which decisions of classification and delivery are based. Thus the abstract and flexible idea of individualization has paradoxically excluded individuals from receiving personalized programmes. In other words the abstract process has been regressed to a traditional and concrete bureaucratic procedure which relates to economic and administratively understood actions.

A further dimension of assessment relates to its role within research. Early research in the field of learning and disability related to experimental techniques and laboratory situations, and a form of control and specificity that may not be entirely conducive to progress at this stage. Action research which is carried out in the field, and arises from demonstration questions and results from consideration of issues that are dealt with in the model put forward, appears more in tune with the goals and aspirations of persons with disabilities. The model helps to provide a format for a line of questioning which can be applied in a sequential manner within the context of the formulated continua.

Another example of assessment in the context of research in the area of information and cognitive processing is the use of assessment in measuring learning to provide more effective strategies of intervention. The work in this area has not yet been subjected to acceptable validation processes, although it is recognized that measuring a process, rather than a product as a basis for assessment, has considerable merit. Feuerstein's clinical evidence does provide some support for this method. The work of Das (1985), and Hallahan and Kauffman (1978) promotes the need for more research in this area.

Another consideration is the multidisciplinary nature of the assessment process. It should be realized that functional behaviours, as observed in assessment, provide a basis for effective interpretation and prescription, but physiological components of the individual's functioning should not be ignored. A medical assessment model is also highly relevant to aspects of treatment. Although a plea has been made for the critical involvement of functional assessment and its application to prescription and intervention, one must not forget the relevance of other types of assessment necessary in the rehabilitation process. For example, within the medical model the orientation of assessment and diagnosis as a necessary precursor to treatment and successful reduction of symptoms is an important component in the treatment of disabilities.

Although functional behavioural assessment has been emphasized, it should not be suggested that other kinds of assessment, which may employ more conventional test modalities, are ineffective. It is the integration of different models which allows for a transdisciplinary approach. Yet in many cases not all assessment modalities are necessary, and assessment needs have to be examined. In many centres a total or comprehensive assessment is provided on a routine basis. This is costly and not always in the client's best interest. If such assessment discrimination is made, criteria for doing this could be developed through this model. For example, regression of behaviour may be due to a variety of causes. If such regression is maintained, if it is very dramatic, or it occurs without social or psychological stimuli which are unfamiliar or stressful, then a medical assessment would be warranted.

Although integration of disabled children into school situations is being carried out and evaluated, this is not occurring in a wide range of programmes for older adolescents and adults, including, and in particular, elderly persons. Here the assessment results are often employed to segregate individuals into what are considered to be groups of homogeneous functioning individuals. The model put forward indicates that, although individuals may show some behaviour in common, enormous variability will remain. Further, individuals oscillate in performance and behavioural changes occur. Thus, even if individuals are put into a group where baselines match at one point in time, very quickly they will be seen, because of behaviour changes, as a heterogeneous group of performers.

The model argues for individual planning and processing. Therefore the idea of putting people together in specific groups on the basis of diagnostic or baseline behaviours would seem as a general rule to be inappropriate. This has relevance for placement in training which we have argued should generally be community- or home-based, and it also suggests that the traditionally accepted differences between various diagnostic groups, such as Down's syndrome and phenylketonuria, may be irrelevant when considering programme planning. The argument may also be applied to other broader categories such as mentally handicapped persons and head-injured, car accident victims.

Assessment techniques

It is recognized that many traditional tests may be viewed as behavioural descriptors, and hypothesis-generators. It is also argued from the model that measurement of behaviour along the rehabilitation continua described is important for baseline assessment if a comprehensive programme plan is to be developed. Behaviour must also be measured in relation to social context and environment.

There are at present a number of assessment techniques, particularly rating scales, which describe behaviour. Examples include the Progress Assessment Charts, the Adaptive Functioning Index and Coping Skills Index. Although these are often used for disabled persons, slight modifications enable their use for elderly individuals. New developments such as the STAR assessment by Guastaserro and Willer (1982) are directed to the assessment of mentally ill persons (Willer and Guastaserro, 1987). But like the other scales mentioned, it deals with a range of behaviours which indicate the importance of social, nutritional and allied areas. However, it is recognized that there are limitations to rating scales. They are largely screening and descriptive devices, and indicate areas where there is a programme lack and areas of delay in client progress. Further assessment needs amongst elderly persons are discussed by Fry (1986).

Assessment is also a requirement in terms of programme evaluation. Many programmes are very poorly evaluated and training personnel frequently do not recognize the criteria which should be employed to ensure the careful selection of programme content. Obviously new challenges are going to occur in this area as computers become heavily involved in the area of rehabilitation (Ryba and Nolan, 1985; Behrmann, 1984). Software is currently being developed, but much of it is poorly evaluated. Briefly the criteria which need to be employed include the number of individuals on whom the pilot project was worked out, the theoretical formulations as well as practical formulations that went into the design and development of the procedure, the type of individuals on whom it has been validated and the extent of average and range of progress obtained by the individuals concerned.

Many agencies are in the process of developing a wide range of their own material. New programme areas are developing such as in leisure time where very formal evaluations of material and curriculum procedures need to become recognized. It has become fashionable in many countries to develop curricula for the education of handicapped persons, yet such curricula, however good they may appear to be, may contain many aspects which have not been fully investigated or assessed prior to their employment with specific individuals. It is only when we ascertain the effectiveness of these programmes that we can ensure that we have a professional base of curriculum knowledge for the area of rehabilitation education.

Further examples of functional assessments that have new and interesting potential for improvement in the delivery of rehabilitation services include the Self Observation and Report Technique (SORT) described by Rintala et al. (1984). The SORT technique, for example, is a specific measure of health status and functioning for physically disabled individuals, and allows greater opportunity to measure their ability to carry out daily activities independently. Information generated by such devices is important in helping people move from hospital and rehabilitation units into home or community programmes. Another area which is beginning to use functional assessment is the field of psychiatric disability. The relatively late development of such approaches in the mental health field has been based partly on a lack of appreciation that adaptive skills are appropriate aspects of measurement regardless of an individual's psychiatric symptomatology or diagnosis. There is sufficient evidence to suggest that functional status is relevant to programme participation and future success, in contrast to the more traditional view of diagnostic categorization of symptomatology. For example, Dellario et al.'s (1984) development of the Multifunction Needs Assessment (MFNA), is an instrument for examining life skills of those diagnosed as chronically and psychiatrically disabled. One of the major conclusions of this research, which has exciting implications in the area of assessment generally, is that the MFNA shows that there is a lack of consistency in functional skills across hospital and community environments, and that chronic symptomatology has only a weak relationship to functional skills. It was also concluded that there is only a moderate relationship between the practitioner's estimates of client functional skills and the client's own estimates of their skills. Furthermore this research suggests that practitioners must have the skills to assess the type and amount of behaviour a client can currently perform and the amount of behaviour required to function in the environment.

A review of some of the contemporary assessment and adaptive behaviour for mentally handicapped adolescents and adults is given by Halpern *et al.* (1981). This publication covers vocational competency scales, tests relating to prevocational information, a wide range of social skills checklists, including survival skills, e.g. street survival skills questionnaire, self-awareness questionnaire, survival in reading, and a wide range of other instruments. This range of material covers many of the dimensions described in the model.

A more recent area of development has been the examination of assessment procedures concerned with behaviour problems or social—emotional functioning, particularly amongst developmentally handicapped persons. Over the years school psychologists have carried out assessment which includes interviews with teachers and parents, self-reporting and monitoring, rating by others, and now more frequently, the use of direct observation in classroom and other situations. The quality of such data requires further research; however, some of the work of Achenbach and Edelbrock (1982), The Child Behavior Checklist, and Adaptive Behaviour Skill by Nihira, Shellhaus and Leland (1975), represent instruments that examine the quantitative and qualitative aspects of behaviour in the psychosocial area. The development of environmental testing procedures, such as PASS, which include evaluation of environment, speak to the need for a comprehensive evaluation.

Considerable work has to be promoted in relation to description of methods for personal programming, examination of personal desire or wishes, and also description of environments in which individuals live and function. Further, individualization of assessment has been developed in the area of leisure (Leisure Functioning Assessment, Possberg *et al.*, 1979) and is developing in the area of 'quality of life'.

The relevance of the model to assessment

The model described, along with some of the developments that have taken place in a variety of areas of psychology and assessment, lead to the view that much more attention must be given to the processes of learning. This is an argument advanced by Feuerstein and many of his colleagues. It is also recognized that assessment must be a continuous process which is related to the continua associated with the model. It is not only continuous, but multidimensional, both in relation to an individual's functioning, and also in relation to an individual's functioning in certain domains of behaviour such as the social area, leisure time and so on.

It is important that new tests be developed in the modalities of tactile, visual and auditory behaviour. A wide range of tests have been developed in the past, but seem either to be contaminated by mixed modality information or do not relate clearly to the actual functioning areas in which individuals learn to perform.

One exciting area that has been opened up as a result of the broader perspective in the understanding of human behaviour has been that of non-verbal measures of communication (Herman, 1981). It might be suggested that once the barriers of conventional testing had been broken practitioners become more aware of the value of non-verbal communication systems, especially for severely handicapped persons. Research has been directed towards manual communication systems typically using hands and other graphic symbolics. Bliss Symbolics and other communication boards or, more recently, electronic devices using computer applications have been developed (Hawkridge et al., 1985). The development of such non-verbal systems of communication opens new vistas for assessment in individuals who otherwise are excluded entirely from conventional or functional processes. For a full discussion the reader is referred to Jones and Cregan (1986).

Assessment and unfamiliar environments

The model provides detail about the effects of stress and unfamiliarity on performance. This has direct relevance for assessment because psychological and allied assessment processes frequently take place in unfamiliar environments with unfamiliar people and unfamiliar materials. If an effective baseline is to be obtained then it is important to measure individuals in situations which are very familiar. This either means going to the environment in which the individual usually performs, and this may be particularly important in relation to certain types of baseline assessment such as those relating to skills that are required in home or community, or it may involve familiarizing people with particular situations so that assessment can then be carried out.

It is recognized that disabled people have to face unfamiliar and stressful environments and testing in these situations or, in replications of these situations, may be important in order to find the effects of such environments on the performance of the individual. This is rarely done with this purpose in mind, yet it is critical to the placement of individuals into new work situations and new homes. The effects of unfamiliarity or stress, for example, on individuals who have become depressed, or the effects of taking individuals who have been disabled and are now returning to work, require that there is a measure of the extent of behavioural regression under these circumstances. Although general guidelines are available, specificity is required. These factors are rarely taken into account in the assessment of individuals.

These same factors are relevant to assessment in other areas which may not be directly behavioural. For example, the ability of individuals to respond to instructors and medical practitioners in assessment situations relating to diagnostic procedures, even of a physical nature, may be influenced to some degree by the individual's familiarity with apparatus, conditions and the requirements. Yet the psychological effects of assessment devices, and of waiting periods in clinics, are not always taken into account.

Transfer and assessment

In the same way that there should be baseline and continuous assessment of a variety of performance processes in a training situation, it is important to measure behaviour change when performance moves to transfer situations. As Das (1985) points out, there are situations of near and far transfer. Mentally handicapped people, and possibly other disabled groups, seem more effective in near transfer, where they apply direct skills to similar situations, but in far transfer environments the nature of tasks changes, so that although transfer is still possible it is more remote from the original situation.

In setting up assessment procedures for measuring transfer it may be necessary to look at the modalities and training continua involved within the proposed model. Thus regression may be expected to occur when transferring to new tasks, and allowance must be made for this. But it must also be recognized that regression is varied, and more complex processes, such as auditory behaviour, are more likely to regress before visual. Thus there must be a means by which each aspect of transfer is measured. At present there appear to be no formal acceptable tests of transfer in the field of disability. The model provides suggestions for the development of such a range of material.

Experience suggests that a variety of transfer situations would be necessary before effective performance could be obtained. The need to provide situations where an individual can learn the skills of adaptation in changing situations is critical, and most rehabilitation centres do not provide this. For example, before attempting to place an individual in employment the effects of different supervision, workshops, peers, and instructions should all be assessed. It must also be remembered that scores obtained on any assessment process must be interpreted in terms of what is to be learned next, for there may be changes in modality, continuum and in content as the person progresses further.

Assessment of staff and environment

It is necessary for those who are carrying out the teaching or training to assess themselves and be assessed by others. This is extremely important in relation to the model because, as indicated, different roles need to be taken by people at different times in relation to any particular client, depending on the stage of development of the individual in training. Thus a teacher may have to be a director, a model, a guide or an assessor. It is therefore important to measure the effectiveness with which personnel carry out such functions. This matter is discussed in a later chapter.

A similar issue arises in relation to environments. The structure and flexibility of the environment are important dimensions in relation to the learning level attained by an individual. Therefore there is a need to develop some measures of environments, for their structure and stability, or their lack of structure and flexibility, are likely to determine whether a particular individual is able to benefit from them. Although there are measures of environment, the type of flexible measures that we have in mind have yet to be developed. Many of the environmental processes for

measuring are at present descriptive of physical attributes of the environment, sometimes social, but rarely psychological. Environments can be modified by the
behaviour of teachers, friends or relatives. Indeed, as indicated elsewhere, recovery
from deprivation may critically depend on the behaviour of persons relevant to
disabled individuals. It is likely that some teachers can perform or teach better than
others in certain types of environment, while other personnel may show a range of
flexibility which we believe may be the hallmark of the field of rehabilitation
education.

Few agencies carefully monitor the amount of time that particular staff spend in
various facets of training. Such measures as amount of time spent in individual
instruction and assessment, group instruction, maintaining records, keeping the unit
tidy and so on, are sensitive measures of the manner in which a particular
programme operates. Not only may they reflect the efficiency of a particular staff
member, but they may also indicate whether the philosophy of an agency is being
put into effect at the front-line level. Obviously an ideal programme in theory, with
adequate materials and curriculum content, will not work effectively unless
adequate staff time is given to individual or group instruction. Unfortunately recent
data (Brown, Bayer and MacFarlane, 1987) suggest a very short period of time
during each day is given to individual training, or even group training, within many
adult rehabilitation agencies. The problem here is that it is not sufficient to measure
the functioning of the individual at specific points in time, but it is critical to
examine the environment and programme procedures that are applied to the individual in order to obtain a holistic understanding of the individual's development. In
order to obtain such information it is necessary to ensure that staff have adequate
knowledge about such processes, and they have adequate time to organize their daily
programmes so that specific needs are met.

It also means that an agency must provide opportunities for the sampling of the
behaviour of agency personnel and examine the extent to which the results match
philosophy and programme requirements. The time available for such activity is
often restricted, and it probably does require the type of management system that
can be provided through the use of computer technology. It is only with printouts
detailing each of the areas described that it becomes possible to have a realistic view
of the total programme-client involvement.

Many of the ecological inventories developed by Lou Brown and associates from
Wisconsin have clearly identified ways in which teacher can examine expectations,
tasks, subtasks and activities within environments in order to plan a useful, functional,
observational checklist regarding student performance. However, these measures,
though useful in describing what is and what would be required in the next environment, do not necessarily look at other aspects of learning structures such as social,
emotional and psychological components required for successful learning.

Agency evaluation

This leads to a discusson of assessment of agencies and their programming, for
unless these can be monitored it will be difficult to see whether particular

individuals can not only survive, but learn, within such environments. In other words there must be a match between the needs of the individuals attending and what is being offered by the agency. Hopefully agencies will be diverse and flexible. However they frequently have a rigid philosophy which cannot be adapted to the needs of particular individuals (see later chapter). Recent data suggest that many agencies for adults concentrate on vocational skills, while individuals need training in social skills. Some agencies state they are rehabilitative in philosophy, while examination of their programmes indicates they are performing as sheltered workshops. The same evaluation concerns relate to home and community environments. For example, many homes do not provide opportunities to learn simple household skills such as changing light bulbs. Unless we know what the individual can do, what skills can be offered in a particular environment, and the extent to which the relevant persons in those environments will provide opportunities for learning and teaching, we are unlikely to be able to measure overall programme effectiveness.

Of course the previous comments relate specifically to facility-based training services. In the 1980s much more consumer-controlled and non-facility-based services will develop, and new challenges will be faced in creating assessment devices reflecting learning experience. This will make it possible to provide more effective structures for rehabilitation.

Quality of life measures

The individualization of the assessment and training approach, particularly using specific environments within the community, gives rise to the question of quality of life and the need to assess this particular area. Quality of life is important to the model at each stage, and becomes more and more important as the individual internalizes structure, because internalized structure means that choice is paramount in the individual's lifestyle. The ability to measure the degree of choice available, and also to measure what it is the individual wants from his or her lifestyle, is critical. At this point a number of quality of life measures are under development (Brown *et al.*, 1986; Cunningham, 1987; Parmenter, 1987).

Quality of life can be measured both objectively and subjectively, and basically refers to the discrepancy between what an individual has attained and what the individual would like to attain. It is also reflected in the extent to which the individual within the environment can gain increasing control over that environment. Two methods have been used to develop measures of quality of life: (1) self-reports by the individual, covering the standard areas seen in the various continua such as social, leisure time and vocational ; and (2) reports made by others who either live very closely to the individual, or in many cases may be parents or spouses. The perception of both groups should be taken into account, for not only are they in one sense a reliability check on each other, they also provide measures of perception discrepancy which form the basis for discussion with the disabled person. This includes, for example, the range of privacy individuals are given, the extent to which they can control their own funds, the extent to which they are seen as needing support, and the degree to which they are being taught to control the environment in which they live.

Quality of life measures an individual's concerns, worries and wishes, as well as providing descriptors of environments in which he or she is trained. The latter includes availability of equipment, the physical positions from which staff carry out individual training, the resources and personal possessions, and the range of space for private and communal functions. All these are relevant to the way in which quality of life is assessed for people with all forms of disability. Many of these are new developments which have not been described in detail but are now being evaluated through a number of centres (see Denham, 1983; Brown, Bayer and MacFarlane, 1985; Blunden, 1987).

The work by Dowrick and Biggs (1983) on the use of visual video techniques and assessment is very important in this context, both in terms of the modification of behaviour (Dowrick, 1978) and for obtaining continuous records. It again speaks to the importance of visual and not just auditory methods of assessment and recording. All of this suggests (a) a knowledge of individual need, (b) opportunity within the local environment and (c) the possible interface between the person and his environment. Finally, it assumes a unique objective assessment, but need not involve normative data, for comparisons with others is often irrelevant.

There is now considerable evidence suggesting that the training offered by various agencies is very different from what parents, spouses or clients actually wish the individual to learn. Recent evidence (Brown *et al.*, 1986) suggests that adults in vocational training centres have an accurate perception of skill attainment and can identify areas in which they have minimal skill. It is corroborated by objective evidence that these centres do not train in the reported areas of deficit. Quality of life also implies a recognition of internal concerns and wishes. The hopes and fears of individuals with disabilities are often not discussed with them either by professionals or family members. A list of concerns noted by Brown, Bayer and MacFarlane (1985) includes concerns over behaviour of trainers to the client or other clients, death or the possibility of death amongst friends and relatives, and issues relating to sexual and allied abuse. It is only when we recognize these concerns that appropriate assessment techniques will be discussed and applied.

The ability that computers have to present certain types of stimulation or procedures in a precise and controlled manner is an important innovation in assessment and training. Computers are also important for comparison purposes in demonstration studies where different procedures of assessment and training may be both calibrated and systematically evaluated by means of computer strategies (see Ryba and Nolan, 1985). Yet the use of computers must be systematically tested and validated along with relevant software packages. The views of the consumer are as important as those of the personnel.

Assessment during placement and follow-up

The model that has been put forward is one of change, and it is recognized that individuals move along a variety of continua becoming more and more flexible as structure is internalized. But it is recognized that individuals regress within these continua when new stresses and problems arise. New issues and problems are likely to occur throughout life, and therefore as external environments change in relation to jobs or communities, or home living, additional supports may be necessary. This constitutes one of the major challenges in the rehabilitation field, for it at once indicates that the process of rehabilitation never ends, and that continuous assessment, particularly at key periods of stress, must be made available so that additional support and monitoring can take place. Without this individuals are likely to fail and return to more institutionalized settings. Minor increases in structure during mild behavioural regression due to environmental change may prevent such breakdown.

This raises some very complex issues about what constitutes rehabilitation, for change and stress, regression and relearning occur to every one of us. Some people, with certain types of physical impairment or mental illness, may not need such support, yet changes possibly make them more vulnerable than non-disabled persons. A distinction therefore has to be made in terms of the service provided. It is important that individuals do not deteriorate to the point where they need comprehensive services, but can obtain resources which are familiar and useful to them at the point when stress occurs. This is an economic investment, and in our view is an ethical requirement within a social service system. In other words our society must consider a comprehensive or a generic service which may involve any of us at different times of our life span.

Management of assessment data over time

The question of the life-long nature of rehabilitation, and the concern for familiar and ongoing services which would be available to people over lengthy periods of time, raises issues for the management of assessment data. How does one maintain useful up-to-date data and relevant information on individuals, that can be accessed quickly by trainers and assessors? Computer management has relevance to this aspect of storage and retrieval, and can make available a considerable amount of information to a variety of recognized personnel. It also assumes high ethical standards of practice and reciprocal recognition amongst the various professional groups. It should be recognized that such a system linked to long-term data preservation is only of full value if the dynamic nature of behaviour change is recognized by those taking part. Otherwise it merely becomes a classification system which aids bureaucratic and rigid decision-making.

Classification

A further theme in rehabilitation which is undergoing radical change relates to our concept of diagnosis and classification. Classification is one of the major structuring processes that man undertakes in order to bring meaning to information that is available to him. Generally such classifications are an attempt to associate underlying processes with one another, and with manifest behaviour or systems, and also provide for links between various sets of data.

The field of rehabilitation has for a long while been based on classification systems which are essentially of medical origin. In more recent years the concepts of intelligence and social functioning have been taken into account in classifying the degrees of handicap amongst individuals. Such a system might be an effective one if individuals maintained their position within such scales, or if they enabled us to segregate individuals from others in society on an effective basis. Unfortunately, or fortunately, neither of these conditions is true, for change and development amongst handicapped persons and the degree of intragroup variability are very considerable. In recent years the writings of Feuerstein (1979) on the one hand, and Stott (1977) on the other, have indicated not only that is change possible, but that we can well mount an argument suggesting that there are no major differences in the principal behavioural structures between handicapped and non-handicapped individuals (Hallahan and Kauffman, 1978). Obviously there are differences in terms of degree. Not everyone would accept such an argument. There are those who suggest that the behaviour of Down's syndrome children is markedly different from other people with moderate or severe mental retardation (Gibson, 1978). To suggest, however, that such differences should be used as a means of classification, or indeed as a variable in selecting different treatment agencies, is probably inappropriate at this stage.

We have developed our knowledge of behavioural systems, so it is now more important to attempt classification on behavioural grounds. This does not negate the arguments put forward by medical practitioners for the labelling systems they employ, relating to genetic or specific clusters of physical symptoms. These have validity in terms of the practice of medicine.

However, this book is not about medical practice, but about behavioural practice, and we must ask the question whether the same type of system of classification has meaning and validity for the practitioner in the broad areas of behavioural intervention. It seems possible that such a system might or might not relate to underlying functions of the central nervous system. In many ways one cannot conceive of a behavioural system being separate from this; on the other hand, alternative arguments come forward. For example, different types of classification may be appropriate for different forms of programme usage. That is, there are different levels of programming and therefore classification relating to this programming will not necessarily have a one-to-one relationship with another system. In other words a medical classification system must not be imposed on a behavioural system with the expectation that it will necessarily provide clear demarcation and direction, e.g. a diagnosis of schizophrenia, while accurate medically, may bear no relationship to where someone should live.

Range of assessment in behavioural skills

It is interesting to note that the more acceptable checklists which measure vocational skills, such as the Mid-Nebraska Three Track System (Schalock, Ross and Ross, 1976), the Progress Assessment Chart (Gunzburg, 1969), the Adaptive Behaviour Scale (Nihara, Shellhaus and Leland, 1975) and Adaptive Functioning Index (Marlett, 1971), conduct observations largely concerned with social skills in vocational situations, and it is these skills which seem to be necessary to successful vocational outcomes (McKerracher, 1984). Unfortunately they are not the most easily measured, trained and practised in other environments or maintained over time.

The wide range of material that needs to be assessed within any rehabilitation programme is obviously varied, both in terms of its range and complexity. It has been suggested that we need reliable and more complex measures, yet here we suggest that the depth of sampling, the precision of the measurements and frequency of the measurements should vary according to need. At times it will not be necessary to have detailed normative data on individuals. In fact we would argue that this is rarely the case, and that such material will only be used under special circumstances. It is also believed that criterion-reference testing will be amongst the most important forms of assessment, detailing baseline and development in terms of attaining goals in relation to specific curricula or programme opportunities. An argument is also put forward for the importance of surveying the needs of the individual, not only by observations of the person's behaviour, but by simple and direct questions to the individual and sponsor.

Concluding comments

Within the assessment process it is important to have an overview of what is offered by a particular agency, both in terms of its philosophy, its actual practice, and application by staff members. We have suggested that the most reliable measures are not necessarily the most accurate measures. For example it seems to us likely, within certain behavioural characteristics, that variability will be the rule of the day. The model that we have put forward in relation to rehabilitation is that stress and new learning, and the application of new tasks and new situations, will result in sudden increases or decreases of performance within an individual. For example individuals who are assessed at the beginning of the day, under familiar circumstances with someone they know, may do very much better than when tested later in the day by someone who is less familiar, or someone who is under stress and is in a hurry to obtain results and conclude the clinical session.

Further, individuals who are in the rehabilitation process face a variety of emotional stresses during the day. An individual who has had to tackle a difficult task in a workshop or school and is then taken to an assessment medium, is likely to show regression of behaviour and perform below his or her average level. That such a result is lower than previous results may have nothing to do with the unreliability of the test, but will be a reflection of the sensitivity of the test. Obviously such performance variability in the behavioural area is likely to be found when dealing with new areas of performance which are subject to variation because of stress factors, or in the field of personality or emotional variables where we still seek reliability. However, by the very nature of the behaviour and the environmental situations variability is likely to occur. Because of this we suggest that the concept of reliability is re-examined in relation to the types of situations in which measurement is taken. The results of the rehabilitation model suggest that variability and change in performance over very short time spans is highly likely amongst individuals who are disabled. Part of this variability not only reflects the difficulties which an individual faces, but may contaminate, to a very large degree, the measures of progress that are being made within a particular area.

Examples are given of how baselines may change over a very short period of time. We advocate the use of multiple baseline measures before proceeding to behavioural intervention. We have already referred to the importance of making some evaluation of the primary and secondary impacts on the individual.

Assessment should be a multi-faceted process. We must have comprehensive measures in all the areas of functioning, for unless we have a profile of the individual's strengths and weaknesses we are unlikely to build effective programmes. It is also important that we measure and assess the transfer process. It is likely that the wider the range of specific skills an individual has within a particular domain, the more likely it is the individual will eventually transfer to new situations. Thus one of the problems confronting many disabled persons is the breadth of baseline of specific skill learning. Non-handicapped individuals, with their broad experience of specific examples, gradually accelerate in terms of transfer. For example, an individual who drives one car may find learning to drive another car difficult. But should an individual frequently rent cars during the course of the year, he or she will develop the skills of learning how to take over a new vehicle. In other words individuals learn how to transfer. It is in this context that the strategies of programme intervention have been developed by people such as Feuerstein, who argues for an assessment of learning potential in relation to problem-solving skills (Feuerstein, 1968; Haywood, 1984). An interesting review of non-intellective factors in dynamic assessment such as the Learning Potential Assessment Device has recently been produced by Tzuriel, Samuels and Feuerstein (1987). However, unless there is sufficient specific skill learning in the first place we believe it is unlikely that problem-solving ability is going to be manifest to a very high degree. In other words the substitution of an instrumental enrichment technique using problem-solving strategies is likely to work best when there is an adequate baseline of specific training in the first instance. We argue, then, not for the substitution of new methods, but the integration of different methods of programming in order to bring about more effective rehabilitation strategies.

The preoccupation that many professionals have with testing out specific methodologies will probably be self-defeating. It seems likely that it is through a combination of methodologies that we are likely to produce a more effective intervention process. It is suggested that the model that has been provided indicating different types of intervention and different needs at different points in time of learning, provides a system through which such processes may be applied. The type of assessment which is used at different stages of the model may be critical in terms of programme assessment and the method of intervention.

CHAPTER SIX

Some neurological and behavioural concerns in rehabilitation

Introduction

This chapter is concerned with aspects of neurology and psychoneurology. It is an attempt to indicate some of the relevant mechanisms which may have a bearing on the processes of behavioural structure and intervention which have been described in the field of rehabilitation. It is recognized that this is a developing area and that some of the arguments are speculative and lean heavily on generalizations from a range of animal studies. Yet one is impressed by the consistency of some of the findings and the parallels in behaviour within the field of disability, including the apparent need for particular types of stimulation and structure to be applied in overcoming deficits in behaviour.

The brain as a sensor

The more complex a vertebrate organ the greater the complexity of stimulation required to ensure its appropriate development. Constant, but varied and simple stimulation is required for muscle development and retention of muscle tone and size. The development of visual and auditory processes is more complex, while the development of the nervous system, particularly at the cerebral level, represents the most complex of processes and, at the highest level, concerns abstract thinking. One important question is to ask whether the brain increases its functioning power as a result of increased stimulation and decreases its power with reduction of stimulation? In extreme conditions (i.e. no stimulation) the central nervous system breaks down. Visual deprivation from birth, in some mammals, has been shown to reduce dendritic growth in the visual cortex (Huttenlocher, 1975).

There are ample psychological and evolutionary reasons to speculate that the central nervous system is dependent on the basic sensory structures and their interaction, and is more susceptible than any other organ to stimulus change. It is the most delicate of our organs and in many ways the most protected. As the most sensitive, it might be expected that it is affected by relatively little change in stimulation, while disturbance in the receptors is likely to have a profound and confounding effect on its functioning.

Like most sensitive apparatus, when its protective devices break down there is major destabilization. It is therefore not surprising that one major phenomenon of central nervous system damage is variability in individual performance—like a compass needle which is jogged and ceases to give a true magnetic reading. The aim of rehabilitation is to find the means of stabilizing behaviour when breakdown or instability occurs. It is suggested that this can partly be done by systematically organizing the presentation of environmental stimulation.

Brain function, environment and change

The model presented assumes an interactive process between brain and environmental structures. It also assumes that both are dynamic structures undergoing change with both developmental and regressive cycles. We have demonstrated, in a variety of ways, the changing flexibility of environmental structures and in psychological terms have represented the changes in self-image and internal cognitive processes and, by implication, affective processes. The model argues for changes in neurological structure, either at a physical or anatomical level, or at a biochemical or physiological level, and the model put forward is dependent on there being such changes.

An early hypothesis

Hebb (1949), with very little physiological or neurological evidence but on the basis of psychological information, argued that some of the phenomena associated with memory loss in instances such as epilepsy, and in other cases of organic damage, could be accounted for by a two-phase learning and memory system. He suggested short-term memory does not involve organic changes within the nervous system, and therefore could be easily disrupted because it is associated with temporary electrical and also biochemical changes. Longer-term memory, he suggested, is associated with actual organic development involving changes in growth and the positioning of dendrites within the grey matter of the brain. To account for the development of learning and memory he posited the concept of phase sequences and reverberatory circuits, suggesting that stimuli, once provided, could set in sequence a series of electrical discharges which could activate, in turn, different neurological cell structures. Repeated stimulation, he suggested, results in the reactivation of the circuits, and with continued and regular stimulation a reverberatory circuit could be established which is continuous and results in the growth of dendrites towards one another, thus facilitating the nature of continuous stimulation.

Although many of the psychological processes described by Hebb could be explained by such a system, very little evidence actually existed to support such a model. The causation of such changes needs to be examined with great care, and this is still an area of some considerable speculation. It is argued, and with some support from biological investigations (e.g. Rosenzweig, Bennett and Diamond, 1972; Goldman, 1975), that environmental stimulation of a social and psychological nature can enhance the growth of the central nervous system and result in an increased network of dendritic endings in both number and inter-dendritic contact. If this is substantiated in subsequent experimental work there may be a valid argument for supposing that the nature of psychological intervention is extremely important in the development of neurological changes. Neurological recovery may take place as a result of this stimulation in individuals who have major central nervous system damage. By the same token it may be supposed that faulty learning strategies could give rise to inappropriate or undesirable dendritic connections. Some support of this view is given by the work of Finger and Stein (1982).

The dendritic changes that occur may be the result of repeated stimulation in a structured, formal and repetitive environmental matrix (Olds, 1975). This is of course consistent with the arguments put forward earlier; namely that rehabilitation processes cannot be haphazard, must be structured and programmes must be integrated with one another over an extensive period of time. It would also seem likely that during the initial phase of learning, or while the responses are being established, sudden regression effects may occur as a result of internal stresses to the organism, or to changes in the external structure of the environment. This may mean a long and structured process to learning, but it is also well known that unless learning can be transferred, performance may be precise yet limited to contextual situations which are identical or very similar to the learning situation. Thus simple but limited instances of rehabilitation occur.

This argues for the development of a structured to unstructured learning paradigm which recognizes the effects of the changing and oscillating structures that continue with the change process. What now needs to be sought is the nature of the more permanent structures which occur as a result of continuous stimulation. Knowledge is required in terms of the extent to which learning is modified by the condition of the central nervous system. It may be supposed, for example that the greater the number of neurons present, and the better the supportive tissue for those neurons, the greater the possibility of rehabilitation, simply because the number of dendritic endings available is very much greater. It may also be conjectured that if the amount of cell damage is considerable, then the growth of dendritic endings during recovery needs to be that much greater, and therefore the rehabilitation process will take a much longer time to occur for required performance to become permanently established. This conceptualization is not in contradiction to the intervention processes that have been argued for preschool children, and particularly handicapped preschool children, where Bronfenbrenner (1976) has put forward the view that long-term and highly structured stimulation, as well as enriching stimulation, is necessary for growth. All three aspects are important because:

1. repetition may establish the nature of permanent change within the brain system;
2. enrichment provides not only for a wider range of stimulus and response bonds to be learned, but learning can take place in a context where transfer is possible, and thus enables the individual to apply his learning in a wide range of systems as in Bronfenbrenner's (1979) description of ecosystems.

The fact that such learning must be highly structured in the first instance reflects the nature of change that would appear to go on within the nervous system. If structure is not present then it is unlikely that effective learning can occur. Thus a limited number of permanent bonds will be established. One would expect that the greater the 'intelligence' of an individual the shorter the time of exposure to extreme structure required. It would seem possible that too much over-learning, too much enrichment and too much structure could also result in limiting individuals, both in terms of an ability to generalize to similar but different environments, and also in terms of obsessive, ritualistic patterns that might develop, thus limiting adaptive responses in other dimensions.

Neurological impairment can result in difficulties in the learning of new material because of mild memory loss, which creates slowness in learning, but otherwise allows the person to function relatively normally (Walsh, 1978). This is consistent with a model which allows for damage to dendritic interconnecting structures through loss of cells. Some individuals, with very small amounts of central nervous system material, appear to function remarkably well (Smith, 1983b). It might be supposed the amount of dendritic contact is such that a variety of complex functions can be maintained. By the same token a lessening of the number of cells will reduce the number of possible dendritic connections resulting in a slowing of mental processes, some memory loss, and a slowness in producing responses, because the number of available circuits is much reduced.

In some recent work the brain has been compared to a muscle function which, if it undergoes repeated stimulation, enlarges its capacity. In this case this is not due to the increased number of cells, but to the number of dendritic connections. In this argument loss of cells can be compensated, at least to some degree, by an increase in the inter-dendritic connections.

As Hagin (1982) has pointed out, central nervous system damage involves a wide range of causes, including punctate haemorrhages, cell body changes, demyelination of the white matter, and localized contusions of cortical tissue. The effects of these traumas may decrease after injury, and Hagin particularly notes the importance of the first three months of recovery, but argues that functional language abilities may continue to improve over a considerable length of time. Once again the impact of cell change and growth would seem to be relevant.

Memory, learning and brain structure

According to Greenough (1978) there is considerable merit in using a model of assimilation and accommodation to explain the storing of memories from a behavioural viewpoint. He argues that there are data to indicate that experience can modify the number and/or the pattern of synapses in the developing brain. Indeed Greenough links the work of Piaget (1952a) and Flavell (1963) from the behavioural side to the biological processes suggested by Hebb (1949). If, as Greenough argues, memories in the form of general pictures of cognitive 'maps' occur, then training for specific events alone is unlikely to be a very helpful process. Further, if part of a map or maps are 'removed' due to a trauma or other kind of central nervous system damage, it is more likely that there will be a recovery process in the brain if there remains a relevant *gestalt* on which to rebuild behaviour. This may account for the sudden gains in knowledge in individuals who become brain-damaged and recover after some considerable period of time. For example, a brain-injured individual who has lost the ability to name parts of a car, or can only give a few names, may be aided in rebuilding that knowledge by referring the individual to the fact that a car has a 'front', a 'middle' and a 'rear'. By using such a 'map' the number of the parts of a car named can be immediately increased in many cases. Despite damage, much of the memory bank may still be present and only certain links have to be replaced. Replacing a burnt-out wire in a car in order for the engine to run again may be an appropriate analogy.

In the field of animal psychology, Greenough (1978) has examined possible differences in dendritic branching in the occipital cortex of rats. He recognizes there is contradictory evidence; however, in explaining the results Greenough notes the possible importance of age and nature of behaviour in adult rats, which he maintains are more fearful and less exploratory than younger rats in a complex laboratory environment. This is exactly the concern that is noted in relation to learning in handicapped persons—namely the unfamiliarity appears to inhibit learning. Indeed, some recent research suggests that many mentally handicapped persons and learning-disabled children decline to make overt responses in audio-reading situations (Brown, 1986c). It is suggested that unfamiliarity may cause anxiety which reduces ability to make anticipatory responses necessary to further learning. If responses do occur which are irrelevant to task expectations, they represent the practising of inappropriate behaviour which leads to the reinforcement and over-learning of non-task-oriented responses. This again may critically underline the importance of familiar environments for the development of learning and in the perception of self as a learner (Zigler, 1966). Furthermore, it does not seem unreasonable to suppose that over-learning of such responses eventually takes the form of changes in neurological structure at the dendritic level.

Greenough also raises the interesting hypothesis that synapses, once formed, do not remain for ever; that is, they tend to break down unless there are processes occurring which enable them to be preserved or maintained. The individual who has undergone a traumatic accident, or is removed to an isolated environment, by definition is deprived of a wide range of stimulation, thus promoting a situation, if we follow Greenough's reasoning, where the breakdown of synapses may occur rather more readily because of lack of a broad pattern of stimulation.

Although work in this area largely comes from animal studies, its possible relevance to human development is important, particularly in the rehabilitation field, and certainly seems consistent with knowledge about rehabilitation at a psychological level. In some experiments, for example those of Valverde (1971), a dramatic increase in synaptic connections has been shown in rodents after stimulation by light. This suggests that stimulation triggers the formation of new synapses. According to Greenough there are an increasing number of synapses in various brain regions with increasing age. But the complexity of the situation is underlined through studies such as that of Resnick (1980) which show that long-term processes, such as long-term memory in a new learning situation, may be disrupted by developmental protein malnutrition. Although there are studies to suggest that RNA supplements to the diet of ageing persons improve their immediate memory, further confirmation is required. There is evidence that the concentration of RNA in neurocells increases when they are repetitively stimulated (Bower and Hilgard, 1981).

Altmann, reported by Gaito, noted that enriched environmental experience results in greater volume and weight of the cortex amongst animals. The results came from a comparison with animals reared in a restricted environment. There is also evidence of greater activity within the cortex under the former circumstances (Gaito, 1966).

Although there is a paucity of data in the human field concerning cortical volume and weight, one early example (1892) which involved a post-mortem examination of a person who was blind, deaf and mute, showed that cortical areas involving vision and hearing were thin and lacked the pattern of convolution found in a normal human brain. The area of cortex devoted to touch had a normal appearance (Rosenzweig, Bennett and Diamond, 1976).

The above indicates some of the detailed interactions that may occur between biochemistry, neuroanatomy and behaviour. One of the messages for rehabilitation is that a multidisciplinary approach must be taken and transdisciplinary professionals must be developed. The rehabilitation practitioner needs to be aware of these interactions.

There appear to be dynamic shifts in development of a progressive and regressive nature within the nervous system over the course of child and adult ageing, and these changes occur at least in part because of environmental stimulation. Change may be dramatic and sudden within the nervous system, as is the case with traumatic brain injury. There is also some evidence that neurological redevelopment and behavioural control is possible, although frequently taking place over a very long time. For example, recovery from certain neurological injuries may take place over several years (Finger and Stein, 1982; Smith, 1983a,b). This is not inconsistent with the type of behavioural changes we have posited occurring in the psychological domain. In Figure 11 these changes are shown as a gradually developing and oscillating function with periods of regression and development. Long-term or major but sudden improvement in behaviour argues for more than transitory change within the nervous system. It may be hypothesized that for the more long-term effects permanent structural and chemical changes have occurred within the nervous system. Nevertheless, it must be recognized that research evidence on organic damage and behavioural recovery shows enormous variation in terms of time and extent of improvement (Rutter, 1983).

Early environmental loss and brain function

In the above arguments it is suggested that there is a link between changes in central nervous system processes at a biochemical and anatomical level on the one hand, and psychological growth and change on the other. At this point it is important to introduce arguments relating to early environmental loss in mentally handicapped individuals. In the case of people born with mental handicaps there is generally a consequent reduction in environmental stimulation and resulting exploration, due either to damage to the sensory system or a lack of development of the motor system. Further, controls of the environment, which often result from parents and professionals who wish to restrict the likelihood of damage to the child, also limit the opportunities for stimulation. However, it has been argued elsewhere, (Brown and Hughson, 1980) that such intervention often constitutes the origin of secondary handicaps. Given the above argument it may be posited that loss of environmental stimulation will help to keep the brain in a disorganized condition, reduce the amount of future organization which would otherwise occur, and thus prevent the full use of existing and available cells with a resultant reduction in the growth of dendritic structures. It is paramount that handicapped persons from birth receive, by modifications to the environment, the appropriate stimulation. This is consistent with an argument put forward by Marlett (1986), for she believes that change should be sought in the environment first, not in modifications to and mediation in the individual. Environmental stimulation can, for the reasons given above, reduce disability.

The argument may be taken one stage further. If environmental stimulation can promote or retard the development of cell assemblies and growth changes in the nervous tissue, then there is a direct link between environmental stimulation— whether social, psychological or physical—and the constructive development of the brain.

For many years it has been argued that it is necessary or desirable to differentiate between brain-injured persons on the one hand, and individuals who have suffered from environmental deprivation on the other. Indeed there has been continuous argument on this particular subject with some effort by diagnosticians to support and segregate the two aetiologies. Soft signs of brain injury such as hyperactivity, distraction and short memory span have been promoted (see Rutter, 1983). Yet in certain of these areas, such as inattention and hyperactivity, other researchers have demonstrated that these effects may be caused by environmental instability and are not simply phenomena of brain injury (Brown, 1964; Robinson and Robinson, 1970). Indeed, many of the children reported by Strauss and Lehtinen (1960) in *The Brain Injured Child* appeared to have histories of adverse environment which could have accounted for attention deficits. It also seems possible that some brain-damaged children do not show inordinate loss of attention processes or increased aggressive emotional responses (Pond, 1961). Here it is argued that there may not be any clear differentiation between environmental damage and its effects, and traumatic injury resulting in central nervous system damage. The effects of social and psychological environment on the development of the nervous system probably do not include extreme pathological damage that can be observed at a macro-level, but they may prevent the development of the central nervous system in an effective and structured manner in terms of the development of dendritic contacts and phase sequences. In effect we may witness, through the administration of psychological tests to disabled persons, a 'brain-injured' or a 'brain-deprived' effect resulting from distorted or inadequate environmental stimulation.

Brain and spontaneous recovery

It has been argued in some contexts that in order to assess the effectiveness of rehabilitation it is first necessary to have baselines against which the value of treatments can be assessed (Goldstein and Ruthven, 1983). Many practitioners believe that the brain has considerable powers of spontaneous recovery. The argument here is that environmental stimulation has to occur and that without it brain development or recovery would have been absent. The differential recovery rates may be associated with certain qualities of the environmental stimulation. People may recover because they are exposed to these qualities. Thus the environment itself provides a rehabilitation medium, and it might be wise to investigate which characteristics in the normal environment promote such recovery. Differential recovery rates may not be due to the differences in the nature of injury, but due to differences in the nature of the personal environment. Rehabilitation must capitalize on the natural aspects of the environment which promote recovery in order to enhance the recovery process. This implies an ethological approach to observation and assessment. It might be wise to look at the features of environment which seem to be important, for it would appear that stability, opportunities for the development of self-image, control of one's own environment, the presence of motivating forces, as well as individuals who can tolerate the slow advances of the handicapped person in the context of decision-making and cognitive control, are highly relevant. Although some changes in environment are occurring (Golden, 1981) it seems surprising that most rehabilitation centres do not underline these positive characteristics of a good, natural rehabilitative environment.

Factors associated with age may be critical in recovery, and evidence is still needed in terms of the extent to which dendritic structures can be modified at advanced ages. Obviously dendritic structures change, and if the above arguments are accepted, change is likely to be greatest when new learning is taking place. Since most new learning takes place during childhood, it might be anticipated that there is greater plasticity on the part of the brain during these early developmental years. Rutter (1983) supports the view that brain plasticity may be restricted by the early adult years. However, new learning does take place in older individuals, and it is the stimulation of such processes which may be critical in developing the recovery of ageing persons. Processes that can be used in this context include the relevancy of stimulation and the bonding of cues. By heightening a particular stimulus it is believed recognition and therefore learning can be enhanced. This is a phenomenon that has been known for some time (Zeaman and House, 1963). However, there may be other underlying reasons why such a process works. By bringing into effect relevant and additional cues, so related neural circuits are accessed, thus helping to bond and stimulate the development of phase sequences and their underlying structures of dendritic development. Of course the involvement of irrelevant cues, such as in a highly distracting medium, could bring too many cell assemblies into play, thus causing confusion and a breakdown of the structured learning for which we have argued. Under such circumstances there may be a loss of dendritic structures with concomitants of stress, frustration and further breakdown.

The arguments produced here underline once again the importance of a multi-disciplinary approach, for we are dealing not only with internal processes of a neurological nature, but with the close interaction of social, psychological, rehabilitative and educative processes, which in turn are thought to bring about changes within the central nervous system. The relevance of all the above to assessment processes in rehabilitation is clear.

Brain—plasticity and recovery

The possibility of central nervous system changes in terms of growth and position of dendritic structures as a result of stimulation appears reasonably well documented. The impact of this on the development of psychological processes is important, yet the area has only sketchily been described, despite the fact that there is a fairly long history of study. There is considerable plasticity in the brain; it is greatest in children, and it decreases over time. It was first documented by Bastian in 1898. In a more recent and comprehensive article, Smith (1983b) notes a considerable amount of evidence suggesting that though plasticity of the brain does decrease over time, nevertheless relearning is possible in adults. He faults a wide range of experiments on recovery from central nervous system (CNS) accidents, arguing that their follow-up periods have been too short. That recovery from major lesions can occur after 3 years following operative involvement has been documented. Unfortunately, many studies limit the follow-up to a 2—3-year period. According to Smith many of the studies show marked cognitive defects amongst the subjects up to the 3-year period, but longer-term research suggests that following the third post-operative year 'rapid improvement with recovery of normal pre-operative levels by the fifth post-operative year' can occur.

Smith also gives examples of major recovery in individuals suffering from severe hydrocephaly at birth. Computerized tomographic scans showed ventricular expansion occupying 95 per cent of the cranium. The extent of recovery in some of these patients appears remarkable. A case is cited of one student who obtained a first-class honours degree in mathematics. A further range of studies quoted by Smith show large increments in cognitive functioning on standard intelligence tests. Many of these individuals were tested 5 and 10 years post-operatively. The surgical operations were for the treatment of CNS damage. There is evidence in the work of Smith that development, associated with the commissures, which may take place over many years, may help to compensate by 'removal of functions from one hemisphere to another hemisphere'.

Walsh and Greenough (1976) underline the importance of environmental conditions in the development of intellectual functioning following premature birth and other early brain insults. Both education and socioeconomic status of the parents appeared to be relevant. Although Smith points out there are a number of variables involved in the situation, it is apparent that the results of these studies are not dissimilar to those of Clarke and Clarke (1960), and Brown (1972) with mildly mentally handicapped people from adverse environments who show, over a long period of time, increases in cognitive performance. Such increases were considerably greater than those of subjects from less adverse environments. In most of these cases there was no indication of brain injury, although residual damage could have been present. These results, considered as a whole, may indicate that the line drawn between adverse environmental experience on the one hand and brain injury on the other is an artificial boundary. It would appear that experience (environmental stimulation involving social as well as educational components) may influence the magnitude of development in brain structures. Alternatively, or in combination with this, maturation as suggested by Clarke and Clarke may play a role. It would not seem unreasonable to suggest that, in the case of individuals deprived of stimulation for environmental reasons, brain structure at the dendritic level may not develop adequately. More stimulation or more structured stimulation may be required. Furthermore, where physical brain insult has occurred such injury may, particularly when the individual is young, be compensated for by an appropriately structured and stimulating environment. The effects of this are likely to be seen over many years. Enriched and supportive environments which are fortuitous during this period (following removal from adverse environment) seem to have a major effect on both the individual who previously lived under adverse conditions and the individual who also suffered insult of a traumatic nature to the brain.

Is it then reasonable to separate brain injury from brain malfunctioning or underdevelopment due to environmental deprivation? Major recovery to the brain can occur. Recovery appears related to the state of residual brain structures, and the nature of environmental stimulation. It is argued that one critical aspect of the environment is the type of structuring that takes place and the level of stimulus repetition applied to the individual, often for a period of many years. In the environmental area of stimulation of mentally handicapped preschool children Bronfenbrenner (1976) and others have suggested that at least a 10-year period of involvement is required. Clarke and Clarke (1976) argue that changes may take place at any stage in life, but are likely to be more dramatic if intervention is started at a very early age.

The importance of these findings falls into several areas:

1. they suggest that it is important to be optimistic rather than pessimistic about recovery from brain injury or adversity of environment;
2. intervention should be early rather than late in life, but recovery and growth may take place at any stage;
3. intervention should be long term rather than short term.

Some additional factors should be added to the above. The quality of the environment, in terms of its status—particularly the structured nature of regular stimulation—is highly relevant if internal (that is, CNS) and new but permanent learning structures are to be developed. Although the nature of this stimulation may vary from individual to individual, for there is a wide range of variability, the data argue for a comprehensive approach to rehabilitation which is much broader than the approach currently applied to specific individuals. It is not a matter just of learning specific skills, but learning strategies of problem-solving through the use of relevant and practical examples.

This leads to a fifth factor; that is, learning experience must be relevant to the individual's practical life. In terms of the training of rehabilitation professionals this is critical, for it suggests that it is important to provide them with knowledge which is generic rather than specific. It suggests that habilitation and rehabilitation are not separate entities, as suggested by some professionals, but similar processes which may differ in degree depending on a wide range of variables. The importance of ensuring that quality environments are present for individuals, regardless of the nature of a client's injury, is critical, for it is seen in these studies that recovery is possible even in severe cases of handicap, and this is associated to some degree with the type of situation in which the individual is performing.

Finally, it is of interest that Smith's arguments for long-term follow-up, in cases of brain injury, are paralleled by concerns in the field of mental handicap where short-term studies prevail. Tizard (1974) advocated longer-term involvement, and Brown, Bayer and MacFarlane (1985) have again underlined the very slow and gradual overall progress that takes place for individuals with developmental handicap. Both fields seem to require that rehabilitation take place over a long-term period if success is to occur.

It may be that there are optimal periods for cognitive development. Certainly Clarke and Clarke (1959) have suggested that the late teens and early twenties are a period where major growth can occur in those who were previously in adverse environments. The Clarkes acknowledge that there is no clear explanation as to why this age period is sensitive, particularly when individuals were removed from adversity some years earlier. They argue for delayed maturation and enrichment of environment. It may be that maturation is another way of saying that repeated and structured stimulation is required over a long period. However it is doubtful whether time itself is critical—rather it is what goes on in that time. Thus attention needs to be directed to the quality and quantity of experience within a particular time frame.

The arguments so far imply that change is gradual. Yet examination of individual growth records of normal children suggests that sudden spurts, plateaus and decrements are more typical (e.g. Honzik, MacFarlane and Allen, 1948). Rutter gives examples of rapid recovery from CNS damage in some cases. Further an examination of both Clarke's and Brown's data on cognitive recovery in individuals who suffered from adversity in environment shows individuals demonstrated increments at different ages and the increments could be sudden and dramatic. Once recovery starts it often seems to continue rapidly. This is consistent with Smith's (1983b) conclusions regarding recovery from brain injury after a 3-year period—recovery once it sets in can be rapid! Brown (1972) also notes that recovery is most common in the least-damaged cognitive area. For example, in a 3-year follow-up study young adults from adverse environments showed greatest gains in non-verbal intelligence and least gains in verbal areas, although their verbal performance discrepancies were at the start in favour of the non-verbal area. Although there may be many possible reasons for this selective improvement, the observation seems logical: it is easier to 'repair' the area with least damage. The observation serves as a warning to those who expect rehabilitation to be a short-term process!

On the other hand individuals subjected to short periods of deprivation often show rapid and spontaneous recovery (Schaeffer, 1963), perhaps indicating that initial effects of environmental damage relate to self-concept and motivation rather than processes or structures which are more permanent. This is consistent with the findings of Hebb (1949) and the cognitive recovery of children from severe but short periods of abuse (Lewis, 1954).

Conclusions

This chapter has attempted to examine some of the parallels between neurological and psychoneurological research on the one hand, and clinical and behavioural evidence within the rehabilitation field on the other. It is suggested that artificial boundaries have been drawn between central nervous system (CNS) processes from a neurological point of view, and psychological functions. At the assessment level it is suggested that many current arguments for brain injury versus non-brain injury are artificial in the sense that environment and CNS interact, and that there are parallels of behavioural disruption which can be caused either by CNS damage or by environmental loss. In most cases an interactive process occurs.

The evidence suggests good reasons why development and change through rehabilitation will be a long-term process, for it would appear likely that major changes have to take place within the CNS. It is likely that much of our rehabilitation is currently set within too short a time frame, and that we should give thought to a considerable extension of time with a recognition that occasional support may be required lifelong. Of course this suggests that individuals who are rehabilitated into the community are going to suffer very severe deficits, if there are not appropriate links between the major rehabilitative technologies and the realities of living in the community. It is also argued that much of what has been referred to as brain recovery may, in fact, be associated with the nature and structure of the environment in which the individual is recovering. Arguments are put forward to suggest that certain types of environmental stimulation may have more impact on recovery than others. It is these processes which should be replicated within the rehabilitation setting and investigated through further research.

CHAPTER SEVEN

Application of concepts to practice

Introduction

This section deals with the application of the concepts advanced earlier, including introduction of new environments, new learning situations, and unfamiliarity of stimulation.

A brief review is provided, followed by a variety of examples from different areas of disability. It should be recognized that the guidelines put forward are simply indicators, which it is hoped will assist the practitioner in developing an effective programme with the client. The complexities of situations and experiences necessitate individualization of programme. The guidelines should help practitioners focus on specific components of practice.

Models and the individualization of programme

It must not be forgotten that the model includes several dimensions, each of which has general facets reflecting historical development and environmental circumstances. The pattern of development within the continua, and the tasks associated with each level, provide examples from which individualized programme packages for specific clients could be developed. It is important to recognize that each continuum runs from concrete to abstract types of tasks and that each level provides opportunities for certain types of experience and development. In one sense the fact that programmes have developed in a certain sequence, such as sheltered and vocational training on the one hand and residential and home living on the other, brings some artificiality to our training paradigms. The application of the model is most useful when a comprehensive knowledge of an individual's baseline of performance is available. We must not lose sight of the fact that we require individual answers based on individual profiles and experience. The model can act as a guideline for establishing likely levels of support and priorities for training. Individuals may progress at different rates in different areas; for example vocational skills may be in advance of leisure time skills. An individual may only have a deficit in one aspect of lifestyle such as home living skills. There is interaction in most cases between all areas of functioning. The individual has to be treated as a whole and therefore assessment, examination and prescription have to be comprehensive. The individual who has problems in the world of work almost certainly is going to have difficulties in other areas of performance, not least because of poor self-image. The individual who cannot obtain work may also have difficulties in terms of motivation and physical stamina. The development of physical attainment, good self-image and positive transfer effects are also critical. The eventual transferability of specific skills to a variety of environments must be taken into account.

In a world where work is difficult to obtain, further recognition must be given to functioning in other areas of performance. It may be necessary to ensure that the individual can function in home and social environments, thus boosting self-image, providing a wide range of background skills and acceptance within the family and home. Obviously the sooner this starts, the better. The point of any model, when discussing disability, is that it should be implemented very early in life; that it must involve, and be understood by, all those dealing with the disabled persons concerned; and it must be applied on a consistent basis until structure is internalized.

Attempting to provide structure in an unstructured environment will naturally prove more difficult. For example, in the school system those who attempt to provide education for individuals with a wide range of disabilities must recognize that intervention needs to take place within the local community or frequent failure will occur. Disabled individuals in classrooms are often asked to internalize many specifics, and then transfer this internalized learning to situations which are remote, unstructured and unpredictable.

Review of model components

The first impact of new stimulation is to inhibit responses, but through gradual familiarization with the environment an increase can be anticipated in the range and frequency of responses. Initially, responses will be gross, then move towards the specific. Learning will also proceed from the overt to covert. There is a continuum of growth from gross to specific, from overt to covert or internalized behaviour. Internalized behaviour is the shorthand of performance. It is rapid and effective but vulnerable to external change.

However, if regression is the rule when an individual is exposed to new learning, a modality shift might be anticipated. For example, if new auditory stimuli are introduced requiring auditory responses the individual may attempt to revert to visual behaviour. If the required response is at a visual level the individual may attempt to respond at a tactile level.

In order to improve learning or reach a higher performance level the practitioner must first interpret signals to the client in simplified, gross and overt dimensions. For example, suppose that an individual is given auditory information for assembly of an item. Many disabled persons will attempt to produce a visual strategy, or at least imagine visual supports to assist in carrying out the task, for in practice it is found that many individuals attempt to ignore auditory information, including written instructions.

If, however, a formal auditory system has been previously established, it may aid in the development of a new visual or motor skill. In order to utilize the auditory process, behaviour will probably undergo a shift downwards as discussed earlier, e.g. learning to use a typewriter often results in a shift from rapid covert thought to overt auditory behaviour (Weber in Woodworth, 1938). In rehabilitation, therefore, it is important to allow for an individual showing this form of regression. Such behaviour should be regarded as normal and merely an attempt to resolve a new and difficult situation.

If efficient learning is to take place it must be structured. There must be careful instruction, and the process of learning how to learn is a critical function within such development. The teacher or instructor must prepare the set for learning in order for the learner to understand when he or she must 'get down to business'. Frequent repetition and many similar examples are necessary in various conditions once the basic task has been learned. Thus the following model seems to be appropriate:

1. *Initiation phase*, responses random;
2. *Initial learning* (primary), the learner selects relevant stimuli and ignores the irrelevant;
3. *Initial learning* (secondary), correct responses are selected but over-generalized—the specific response is applied to a class of stimuli rather than a specific stimulus;
4. *Initial learning* (tertiary), the response is restricted to the specific stimulus.

Selection of learning tasks

Once a task can be performed the learning process is often, but erroneously, seen as completed. Even if an individual programme plan is employed the end goal is often a specific activity. The elderly person who has made a basket in occupational therapy, or the mentally handicapped person who has completed the assembly of a toaster unit, have learned specific skills, and this is correctly regarded as progress. But the next stage of learning is overlooked. Learning has to be applied to new situations or new, but related, tasks. First transfer is near, i.e. related activities, but when change of situation and wide variation in task occurs, far or distant transfer is set up (Das, 1985). This transfer must be carried out in a stepwise fashion (Gold, 1973).

A wide learning base with a range of similar activities practised in a variety of situations will help to promote transfer, but such variation must not be introduced too early in the process. Also, the procedures adopted by Feuerstein (1979) for problem-solving are possibly effective methods of promoting transfer. Conscious behaviour in the learning situation and how one 'looks at a problem' should aid in generalization from one situation to another. Thus encouraging an individual, for example, to imagine his or her position in a given space and asking whether an object is to the left or right, in front or behind, should help the process of internalization and problem-solving.

Feuerstein has proposed the development of a problem-solving technique called mediated learning. He argues that by teaching individuals how to solve problems one deals with proximal causes of mental retardation. In one sense this is very similar to the concept of secondary negative impact. The important point about

Feuerstein's model is that it teaches individuals how to deal with problems. The work of Feuerstein is only now undergoing major experimental examination. While the general paradigm is a useful one, it needs to be placed in the framework of a model. It is important that problem-solving techniques are placed within certain modalities and are sufficiently structured that transfer is enabled. The problem at the present time is that neither handicapped persons nor people of average ability transfer very readily to new types of situations.

Once this need for transfer is recognized it becomes apparent that selection of the original task is crucial, simply because some tasks have greater community, social or survival value than others. A task which occupies the time of an individual serves a limited goal. A task which the individual enjoys may serve a wider need, but a task which enables the individual to master environmentally, practically and person-ally relevant behaviour has direct relevance to his or her rehabilitation into society. This evaluation must be applied to the teaching of basket-weaving, toaster assembly and the range of tasks which are common in vocational training settings. Experience suggests that many rehabilitation agencies take what tasks they can get while many hospital departments rely on traditional occupational therapy activities. It is hardly surprising that the clients often do not see the purpose of the task or, at times, may be resistive to involvement!

Although there are exceptions, most clients wish to work on activities which give them environmental control in areas which they regard as valuable. Thus a child who is emotionally disturbed and has a learning disability in reading may wish to learn to read. Play therapy, which may be recommended as a means of dealing with what some may regard as the secondary emotional impact, is 'reading-task irrel-evant'. Gradual control of the reading situation through mastery of skills brings reward and heightened self-image, and more time for play. This is not to say indirect therapies are unimportant, but to argue for a much closer examination of what we teach, and why we believe particular tasks are desirable.

Need for various environments for learning

Not only is there a need to consider carefully the series of tasks used in rehabili-tation. Some thought also has to be given to the type of environment in which learning takes place. It is important, particularly in the early stages of recovery and training, that individuals remain in a stable and familiar environment. Wherever possible a supportive home environment should be available, but it may also be necessary to remove some of the stresses and irrelevant stimulation within such an environment. It should be noted that research (McKerracher, 1984) suggests that personal adjustment and vocational success have a direct and positive relationship to family solidarity. It is also important to recognize that the environment used should generally be where the task is normally carried out. For this reason it may be necessary to personalize environments; that is, individuals should be able to familiarize themselves with an environment and demonstrate they can move around it easily (e.g. location of facilities, exits, work stations) before undergoing intensive training within the environment.

At times it may be necessary to reconstruct environments so that individuals can learn in a formalized controlled setting the types of skills that they need to use. Unfortunately the more different the actual learning environment from the real place where opportunities will eventually be available, the more difficult and problematic becomes transfer. This is one of the reasons why environments for rehabilitation, which are remote from the area in which the individual functions, are less adequate and probably rather more time-consuming in terms of learning. For example, mobility training for visually impaired persons should, wherever possible, take place in an environment which is the same as, or similar to, that in which the individual is likely to operate (Brown, 1985), even though it may be important to implement initial training in a more simplified environment to ensure that learning is as fast and effective as possible and thus more rewarding to the individual. But the issues of familiarity and transfer raised earlier must be considered. Unfortunately, in many countries mobility training for visually impaired persons is only given in a few urban centres, because of the low incidence of visual impairment and a belief that centralized training is more economic. This raises a number of management and design questions which are dealt with elsewhere.

Application to learning environments

What are some of the other applications of the model examined? Does the model provide us with a means of anticipating some of the more generalized behaviours that may be expected to occur under a variety of rehabilitation situations? With such knowledge can rehabilitation procedures be planned more effectively in order to produce less stress and promote better adaptation or more efficient learning?

In a number of instances modification of the environment may have major implications for primary learning situations. This is extremely important to the psychologist, educationalist, social worker or behavioural worker within any treatment or education facility. Indeed there are also situations where an individual is undergoing physical procedures such as dental surgery, or physiotherapy, when a knowledge of these implications may also be important.

It is known that children adapt more readily to temporary loss of a parent if they remain in a physical environment which is familiar to them. It has also been recognized for some time that children improve more rapidly after physical trauma if a parent is present with them during a period of hospitalization. When parents are not present, withdrawal behaviour and silence may result. With parents present less regressive behaviour may involve crying and shouting but the child, like Harlow's monkeys, will then begin to explore and adapt to his or her new environment and deal with the strange surrounding stimuli. In other words, when children are put under stress a range of behaviours occur.

In these situations a U-shaped curve is postulated, with quiet or low response emission typifying different underlying mechanisms at each end of the curve (see Figure 13). When environment or task is familiar the individual will tend to choose a low-key response mode typified by high attention and smooth yet minimal responses. Minimal means the most effective level of response to maintain control of the environment. Strangeness in the environment increases the grossness of response as well as the range, while complete unfamiliarity tends to inhibit responses. A basic rule can be generated from such situations: in any situation of stress or new learning where some change in environment has to occur it is important to keep as many familiar structures in the environment as possible. Environment refers to physical, psychological and social stimuli.

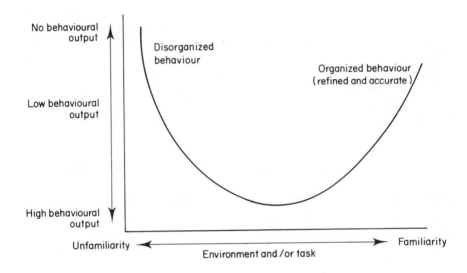

Figure 13. Suggested relation between familiarity of stimuli and observed behaviour.

The argument for familiarization of environment where stress occurs now becomes readily apparent. Thus the elderly woman who has to be taken from her own home because of deterioration of behaviour is unlikely to improve, but to regress further, in new surroundings in an old people's home or hospital. This regression can be modified to some degree by ensuring that increased and familiar structure is involved within the new environment. For example, the presence of some personal possessions and familiar people such as a loved relative, both day and night, over an adjustment period is likely to be highly effective. Wandering behaviour may occur, but can be reduced by referring the individual to concrete and stable cues such as major building structures but not particular staff or room numbers (Hussion, 1981). The same situation is seen when a handicapped individual is required to adapt to a new job, or a first job after initial training in a rehabilitation agency. At such times clients deteriorate in their behaviour, and level of work often deteriorates in quality and volume. The individual is likely to reduce behavioural output and in persons with epilepsy, for example, seizures may also result. The latter example suggests that although external behaviour may be reduced, internal activity may increase, although this is likely to be disorganized rather than organized. To place disabled people in a new situation (e.g. new employment) effectively it is necessary to bring performance above the minimum threshold, because skills tend to deteriorate for a while once the individual is in the new situation.

Indeed to a greater or lesser extent everyone experiences this phenomenon. Change of home from one place to another, or one job to another, results in the personal experience of not being able to remember where items are placed, being unable to recall words which are normally within our vocabulary, names of people, dates, etc. Further, this phenomenon also occurs when individuals return from vacation, for there tend to be problems in establishing basic activities (e.g. difficulty with names, spelling). Other examples include use of new instabank units, travel to foreign countries, and redesigned income tax forms. These are all common environmental situations which cause regression in behaviour, and for which there are compensating strategies to enable an individual to adapt.

Thus at a macrolevel there should be interest in the behavioural signs shown by people under all conditions of stress. For somebody like this who perhaps has lowered self-image, who is possibly aware of limitations or deterioration, placement in an environment, where they find it even more difficult to perform, often accelerates the process of deterioration. This is observed with many disabled persons, but has been particularly noted with visually impaired persons (Jones, Lavine and Shell, 1972), especially those who have recently lost their sight and are elderly (Negrin, 1983). This is consistent with the model described because loss of the visual modality greatly reduces the ability to rely on familiar information. Regression is expected to be considerable because there would, according to the model, be a need to re-establish a baseline using tactile stimulation followed by bridging mechanisms to auditory stimulation. Such a jump across modalities is exceedingly difficult, and probably accounts for some of the stress and self-image problems encountered in mobility training. The successful individual will make use of variation in sound patterns to locate objects in space. Some recent aids capitalize on auditory feedback (e.g. laser guides). However, it is important to commence using these when an effective and stable baseline has been attained and self-image is sufficiently high to enable training to be successful.

It is therefore incumbent on all who work in rehabilitation education to increase familiarization with the environment. This may mean leaving a specific time just for orientation to new situations. Sometimes a period is even required to become familiar with old situations because impairment means that the formerly usable cues cannot be employed. The old environment has become, in effect, unfamiliar.

There may be instances where the opposite is required; that is under certain circumstances unfamiliarity of environment may promote greater stability. A highly distractible and disturbed individual who is hyperactive may, when placed in strange or unfamiliar circumstances, show reduced behavioural output. Thus the person becomes more manageable. For example, a young male with epilepsy showed hyperactive and physically abusive behaviour in his vocational training unit. Such events occurred regularly, and generally after he had been within the unit for about 30 minutes. A psychologist plotted the time and frequency of outbursts and then set up a schedule whereby the individual changed units on a 20-minute schedule. Thus new and unfamiliar environments were used to dampen behavioural output. Reward was given at the end of every successful 20-minute session by unit staff and the psychologist. The number of unit changes was gradually reduced and duration in each unit increased. This programme was successful. It capitalized on two learning principles: (1) reducing negative behavioural output through unfamiliar stimulation which led to (2) an ability to reward the individual for satisfactory behaviour. The example shows how the principles of the model may be used to advantage when an attempt is being made to remove aberrant, overactive and disturbed behaviour, and establish more acceptable response levels.

The process of familiarization to new environments is particularly relevant to developmentally handicapped persons. Because of mental and/or physical disability they are often protected, and at times over-protected, by those around them. Such individuals are often sent to training centres or sheltered workshops primarily for care, with parents specifically requesting they not be trained. If training occurs parents may become concerned and resistant to the greater socialization of the individual. For example parents may say 'we cannot allow him to go on the local bus system because he may get lost', 'we cannot allow her to go shopping in case she is picked up'. What is not realized is that if a training hierarchy of the type discussed is carried out, by means of small stepping stones an individual can learn to deal with such situations. Individual clients are gradually introduced to unfamiliar aspects of the environment and taught how to deal with them. Apparent confusion and incompetence mainly occurs when such individuals are suddenly 'dumped' into new situations where regressed and maladaptive behaviour is to be expected. The behaviour shown is not abnormal, and represents an expected response when the learning steps are too great. Very young children frequently behave this way. Such behaviour is only seen as abnormal when the individual is older. Most non-handicapped older people have learned to cope with such circumstances through performance strategies which may include avoidance.

The protection argument is one that predominates in the care of disabled persons, because professionals themselves are often concrete in their thinking. It is also understandable that many parents react in a protective fashion, for the training or education of their child may represent changes for themselves with unknown consequences, which give rise to unfamiliar challenges and increased anxiety. Parents may themselves show temporary regression in behaviour in these circumstances. The same phenomenon is seen with adult offspring caring for an elderly relative, and later we shall discuss the same behaviour within professional staff.

It is essential that parents or sponsors are provided with examples, so that they can understand what occurs behaviourally under these circumstances, and how such behaviour can be effectively controlled while promoting growth within a structured rehabilitation programme. Individuals who are prevented from going to town or travelling on a bus to shop on their own, are being physically protected. They are removed from the obvious signs of danger, and risk is not permitted to occur. However the psychological variables which promote learning, and the social interactions which are necessary to improve level of performance, are also removed. Thus lack of psychological growth is promoted and inappropriate forms of behaviour are reinforced. Such inappropriate behaviour, if over-learned, is likely to generalize to new situations. This type of deprivation characterizes the secondary impact of disability discussed under assessment. Unfortunately such situations can result in further behavioural regression, thus confirming the worst fears of those who work with the individual.

It is important to ensure, when positive learning is encouraged, that the environment is bolstered with firm structures to enable the individual to cope. A detailed example of this is provided by Hughson and Brown (1975) within a bus training programme for severely mentally handicapped young adults. Familiarization of the major aspects of the task was carried out including site visits, travel with a staff member and visual slides which could be examined and discussed within a familiar unit. The process was individualized so that each person learned his or her own house-to-agency route. To begin with routes which involved bus changes were eliminated. Once familiarization with aspects of bus stop, bus identification, and fare payment had been dealt with, the individual travelled with a staff member or familiar volunteer, with the individual carrying out all the necessary interactions. When this had been repeated successfully to criterion the individual carried the journey out alone, but a staff member followed by car to ensure the individual did not get lost. All of this worked smoothly—the use of familiarization techniques, small steps and visual teaching processes with tactile prompts (e.g. hand on arm to stop or remind) and gradual withdrawal of prompts and internalization of the structured training programme—with one exception. One parent found the process sufficiently stressful that he continued to follow the bus in his own car! Rehabilitation must take the stress factors impinging on other family members into account.

A paradigm is thus available for the development of new learning situations, which can apply across a wide range of behaviour. This paradigm assumes the use of baseline assessment. It is absolutely essential to know how far the individual has proceeded, what opportunities he or she has had in the past, and which aspects of the task he or she can deal with. Such an assessment cannot be carried out on a global basis, but must be directed to the measurement of a variety of specific performance attributes. This is particularly relevant when assessing performance in complex social situations. In the bus training example it was necessary to observe whether individuals could discriminate which side of the road they would locate their bus and whether they could discriminate between different buses. It is necessary to recognize what the individual knows and can do, but it is equally important not to ignore what cannot be done or the level of deterioration that has taken place. An individualized learning situation, where adequate supports are employed to minimize regression effect, can then be designed.

Confused behaviour is likely to occur when the individual is confronted by new stimuli. An individual, particularly a disabled person, is unlikely to know how to respond, or what to respond to, in terms of a new pattern of stimulation. It is important to provide directional and heightened cues in the new situation. The reader will remember that regression may mean that the client has fewer words available than normal, so it is important to cut out a range of auditory stimulation and use visual modelling.

Such ideas are not new; what is new is the idea that this information can provide a paradigm with general implications for the behavioural rehabilitation field. Goals must be specified and specific, and stepped goals for the short and long term are needed in very concrete format as itemized in Martin and Pear (1983), and Marlett and Hughson (1977). Long-term goals must be established, for the aim will eventually be to internalize the behaviour, so that the individual may perform appropriately regardless of whether the trainer is present or absent, and regardless of changes in the situation. Responses should be taught so that they are adaptable to new situations. This particular component raises the nature and role of self-concept, motivation and internalization of behaviours.

Application of a model

The following represents a series of examples which illustrate the use of a model in providing guiding principles for understanding behaviour in the broad field of disability and considering possible programme strategies. It is stressed that the components of the model are well known, though not generally applied. What is new is the organization of the items to form a rehabilitation model. Much of the model is summarized in Figure 10 (see Chapter 4) and will serve a wide range of practitioners. One of the advantages is that individual practitioners no longer need to know the full range of research data that forms the basis of the model. From the model they may devise a range of assessment and programme tools in order to attempt to deal with behaviour of one kind or another. This form of shorthand is essential if rehabilitation is to be effective and bridge the research to practice gap.

Physical illness and behaviour

Let us take the example of an elderly man who suffers a traumatic accident involving his central nervous system. Because of the accident he is taken to a hospital unit and provided with care and treatment. In terms of the model it is argued that this elderly gentleman, even if he had been taken to a hospital prior to the traumatic accident, would have regressed in his behaviour because of the new environment in which he is placed. What form might that regression take? In an elderly person certain types of deterioration processes are occurring. Motor skills are less effective than at an earlier age, the ability to learn and remember new events and to process such information is also restricted. The cues which constitute recognition are missing or confusing, thus interfering with basic memory processes. He sees things less easily and reaction time has increased over recent years, and he fears change and deterioration (Fry, 1986). In general, problem-solving abilities are less effective than during an earlier age. Within a new environment (a new bedroom, new food delivery, new people), with people functioning in a professional capacity, and not responding in the socially accepted ways of his familiar environment, certain behaviours are likely to occur. First he will be very slow at learning the new regime. He will have fewer words available to him than in his own environment. The words available will be more concrete and less accurate, and his reaction time will be slower. Therefore to visitors he will seem to be somewhat more restricted than previously. If, prior to the hospitalization, he had a motor tremor it will now be greater, and he will probably be preoccupied with visual and tactile processes which were less obvious within his home environment. This is partly because he is exploring his new environment, but to do this his behaviour must regress. It is likely that quirks of personality will be accentuated under these conditions, although these may not be readily apparent to begin with, because his behaviour has reduced in terms of output. Thus if he tended to be rather aggressive at home he may now seem rather subdued. Under these circumstances behaviourally he may seem improved. This is a common phenomenon. In new environments many otherwise aggressive or disturbed persons appear tranquil. Staff who are new to the individual may doubt the previous reports of agitation, or aggression, or depression or delinquency. It is perhaps important to stress that staff should observe carefully, but combine the information with reports from previous situations. If there is a difference it is probably not due to error, but may be due to a change in environmental circumstances.

On the other hand much of the behaviour described above is associated by many people with permanent deterioration. Such behaviour is taken as a sign that an individual is less capable of functioning in his own environment because he shows deteriorated performance in the new environment. If the amount of stress is increased behaviour will regress even further. If he also suffers some form of traumatic injury it is likely that much of the behavioural regression, which is initially of a temporary nature, will increase in magnitude and become more permanently established. The interaction between the traumatic physical state and the new environment complicates the issue, and the interaction causes further regression of behaviour. Thus the impact of the two conditions is probably greater than the sum of the two independently. Although we are beginning to gain some understanding of these types of phenomena and their interaction, we still do not recognize them as natural processes, nor do we take sufficient steps to circumvent the difficulties.

If we accept the model of regression we must argue that it is much better, whenever possible, to treat an individual within his home environment, despite the fact that this could give rise to a wide range of stresses to others in the environment. Some assessment of the stability and resilience of other persons in the home environment becomes critical. Further, the availability of a sound health service which can provide support within the familiar environment is highly desirable. Under these circumstances what is familiar and well known helps to provide a necessary and structured environment. It encourages the re-establishment of learning, increases recall, and generally stabilizes the individual. In short, it should lead to an optimum level of performance.

Grief and depression

Regression may occur due to specific deterioration of physical structures of the body or social and psychological stress. Deterioration is likely to be suddenly exacerbated when new and sudden psychological and social trauma occur. The model explains why, when there is a death of a relative or a very close and loved person, an individual who is already disabled or suffering from other stress may now deteriorate to a much greater degree. Self-image is damaged and the normal and familiar supporting structures of the environment disappear. The individual regresses to simpler verbal behaviour and typically in grief situations visual and tactile behaviour results. This is a natural phenomenon and therefore presumably should be regarded as a necessary psychological mechanism to deal with a disrupted lifestyle. It is part of the method for overcoming stress. In the example given, where the individual is already suffering from physical and psychological stress, the loss of a loved person is likely to have a major impact on physical structures because they are already in critical condition.

The model suggests that the grief process is a natural phenomenon which should be accepted since it is part of a normal process of regression which helps the individual gain control of the environment. Frequently we do not allow such processes to take place. Further, when working in the rehabilitation field we may not take into account the effect of such stresses on the rehabilitation process which needs at such times to involve increased support and structure.

It might be appropriate at this point to indicate that the same model leads to the suggestion that depression is a natural phenomenon which may represent an adaptive and stabilizing process (Costello, 1976). It could even be called 'healthy' in the same way as flesh wounds require blood clotting and the formation of scabs. Western society frequently does not accept such a view, and often takes active steps to prevent the signs of depression. An individual who becomes depressed is likely to show regressive behaviour for a number of reasons. First, self-image is dramatically damaged and forms part of the constellation of problems associated with depression. With reduction of self-image, regression to much earlier forms of behaviour tends to occur. There is interplay between earlier and later modes of behaviour which may result in bizarre characteristics of disturbance. An individual with depression is also likely to show regression from auditory to visual components. Depression is likely to reduce the range of words at the individual's disposal, and much of the person's verbalization will be in concrete rather than abstract terms. Severe depression may be expected to take the individual into a tactile area which is frequently observed with rocking and stereotyped tactile phenomena—e.g. finger-tapping. There is likely to be a need to touch and stroke objects. Ritual displays, in which tactile behaviour forms a dominant theme (e.g. tapping an object several times, not walking on the lines) are often part of the characteristics shown in obsessive behaviour.

Much of the depressed person's behaviour will become gross rather than specific. Motor behaviour will begin to break down and fine motor behaviour is likely to be imprecise and slow. Social requirements can only be met if more overt behavioural supports at earlier developmental levels are utilized. Weeping and irrational statements may be anticipated, and those around the person need to provide accepting support and understanding of such behaviour. The model enables us to see depression not as a discrete and aberrant form of behaviour, but as part of the behavioural continuum along which human beings function. Indeed to know precisely what behaviour and its sequence of development an individual may demonstrate would enable us to predict, in general terms, what particular symptoms will be shown in any specific person suffering from depression. Depression, whatever its cause, is *not* simply abnormality of behaviour. It is part of the individual's developmental repertoire.

The model becomes a blueprint or guide to the behaviours which an individual may show under certain circumstances. The individual's genetic properties and his or her environmental experiences will determine the precise behaviour shown. This is consistent with the ethological conceptualization of the model and the behavioural continua. The model also provides a guide for correcting the behaviour. If there has been extensive deterioration of behaviour, with resultant loss of self-image, the environment remains the major area for rebuilding it. When individuals become stressed or depressed environmental structure needs to be increased. Removing structures and allowing open-ended behaviour to occur will tend to result in further regression and the appearance of non-directed behaviour (i.e. the client is 'confused').

Current health and social services dealing with this kind of breakdown tend to reduce the natural and familiar structures, and replace with unfamiliar environments, plus arbitrary authoritarian direction, which on its own further reduces self-image. Few mental health services involve the delivery of services which have as their prime locus the familiar home, family and/or work environments. Mental health treatment generally involves taking individuals into clinics, hospitals or other mental health institutions, often away from their home environment. The individuals are returned home when they appear cured. Yet according to the model it is expected the individual will regress once again when they return home, if the stresses in the original environment which caused reduction of self-image are still present.

This argument may appear contradictory. Using the model as the blueprint it is argued that familiar environments should be retained wherever possible, particularly those aspects which are supportive. But in the situation described the negative aspects of the familiar environment are stressful. Thus the overall environmental picture does not provide a supportive structure. The practitioner must analyse the pros and cons of the familiar or unfamiliar environment and recognize where the greatest difficulties lie—in the stresses of the unfamiliar environment or the stresses in the poor structure of the familiar environment. If the reader examines Figure 8 (see Chapter 4), it will be noted that stress reduces self-image and requires greater external structure in the environment. This may imply using an unfamiliar environment while restructuring the familiar one. Professional personnel must become involved directly within the home and living environment of the individual, if they intend to effect major changes in the performance of the individual concerned.

So the model argues for changes in mental health treatment, an argument that takes us away from hospital care. Some will assert that modern mental health services do not remove the patient from the home unless it is necessary. Out-patient and day hostel services are available. Home intervention has at times occurred. However, the model provides a rationale for applying structured home and community intervention on a regular basis. It is the environment of home and work which contributes to and then maintains disturbance. It provides the stimuli and reinforcement which produce abnormal learning. The restructuring of that environment is essential in such a way that former inappropriate learning can be disrupted, previously established effective learning returned, and new learning introduced. Thus one begins to change the functioning pattern of the individual and also the structures within the family itself.

The model underlines the necessity for treating the family, not just the individual who is suffering problems, but treatment here is perceived as a process of restructuring the environment so that responses and finally overall behaviour are remodelled. This can only be done by observation, then direct and accepted intervention within the individual's own environment. The point is that we are not necessarily dealing with mental illness, but with maladjusted and regressed behaviour. The individual and family must internalize the process or structure and become the architects of environmental change (Tymchuk, 1979). This concept of internal and personal restructuring is seen as a stepwise process in the model with periods of development and regression. The process has much in common with the approach of modern family therapy (Hansen, 1983) and recognizes the importance of the family ecology (Bronfenbrenner, 1979).

Yet family therapy often takes place outside the home and involves largely verbal interchange. We suggest that verbal attempts at modification may, on their own, not be sufficient because of the regression involved. Visual and even tactile components are also necessary (Herman, 1981), and the use of video techniques and familiar places have an important role to play within this system.

Mental handicap

In the field of handicapping conditions the importance of family and environmental intervention can be seen clearly. Mentally handicapped adults are often referred to special services for difficulties in the areas of performance and self-image. In some cases they have been functioning at severely retarded levels of intelligence. In one particular example, in our experience, the parents declined to attend an agency for conferences, indicating that their child was unable to learn, as she was now a young adult, and all they required was care of her during daytime hours. Because of this, and our judgement that progress could only be made if intervention involved the family and their attitudes to their child, two staff were asked to enter the home environment and develop a training programme within the family. The staff were asked to model training processes so that the parents could subsequently take over. The task chosen in this particular case was to teach the young woman how to wash her hair, and this was carried out over a period of approximately 10 days by one member of the staff. This task was selected because the mother indicated that she spent a lot of her time dealing with activities for her daughter, and she quoted this particular task as an example of why she was unable to leave her daughter and could not take a job. On the successful completion of the task the mother indicated that, if the young woman could learn, then why could we not teach her more tasks, thus enabling the family to function more effectively. This was done, and included shopping, use of telephone and other practical activities. We are convinced that no advance could have been made in this young adult's programme, and certainly not this rapidly, unless a programme had been set up within the home environment. The outcome was a dramatic change in terms of attitude, both within the family and within the individual who gained a wide range of new skills. The client became more assertive and obviously built a better self-image.

The account is a clear example of use of the model in terms of concrete demonstration, tactile and visual training, both of which represent a high level of external structure within the familiar home environment. The aim was to produce a change in learning characteristics plus improvement in self-image. Through repeated example the individual gained increasing control of the environment, and in turn reduced the amount of parent control and structure within the home. The client was provided with a means of gaining personal control with the internalization of structure, which could then be employed in new situations.

Examples from the field of counselling

There are a number of instances where counselling is employed in an attempt to overcome difficulties within the mental health or allied fields. Counselling techniques are used, for example, in the field of delinquent behaviour (Romig, 1978). Yet research workers are generally agreed that the various treatment regimes often have poor results with delinquent persons who have come from adverse environments, particularly where there are unstable or poor parental models (Robins, 1966). This is consistent with the arguments we have put forward, for the individuals concerned are for the most part functioning at a very concrete verbal level, and under stress and regression they are likely to act largely within visual and tactile modalities. The model suggests a more basic form of therapy is required, and that counselling or allied therapeutic approaches, when employed, should involve visual imaging and reference to tactile and kinaesthetic behaviours as suggested by Michenbaum (see later). The importance of a relevant or meaningful environment, in which the child has a clear role with opportunities to develop control over this environment, is important for self-image and control of inappropriate behaviours.

The field of counselling has grown phenomenally over the past 30 years. Gunzburg (1960) advocated the use of counselling with severely retarded persons. The work that he cited gave some evidence of success. However, our model suggests that some further guidelines might be put forward. For example, the use of tactile and kinaesthetic references within the language that is employed, and the use of self-imaging might be very helpful. Certainly amongst mentally handicapped persons visual strategies are commonly employed (Landino, 1979), and self-imaging is recommended by Michenbaum as a technique to control various behavioural disturbances in individuals. There is also considerable evidence, such as that of McLeod and Brown (1976) indicating that in verbal encounters clients remember much of their own statements, but relatively little of the counsellor's. This would be expected when the range of client language behaviour is somewhat restricted. It is important for a counsellor to recognize different levels of interaction when dealing with different types of clients with varying levels of baseline performance. The counsellor must also be aware that regression may mean that the individual has some difficulty, no matter how cognitively able, in attaching abstract concepts to relevant aspects of the situation, and that too high a level of verbal involvement may result in further regression. Flexibility is an important component in counsellor style (Herman, 1981) and may help to assist in devising and modifying counselling options. Allowing clients to describe content in their own words, or repeat counsellor comment in their own ways, helps to clarify level of comprehension and encourages internalization of the process by clients.

A similar situation is seen in relation to counselling in physical rehabilitation where an individual returns to the work environment. Accidents frequently occur in the semi-skilled and unskilled workforce. Such employment involves a large amount of movement, and the effects of back injury or other accidents are likely to mean that counsellors will advise sedentary occupations. In many cases this does not work very well. Sedentary occupations often involve a considerable amount of verbal activity, whereas the individuals involved have had a work life largely in the non-verbal domain. The effects of the accident make the individual even further remote from activities of a verbal nature, because of regression and stress that have been involved. There is therefore some reason to hypothesize that such individuals would not readily function in many sedentary jobs. It might be better for him or her to be rehabilitated first via non-vocational aspects of living—namely in family, community and leisure time areas. Such areas can involve a large element of non-verbal, or low-level, or restricted verbal interaction. If such methods are employed and effective behaviour established, then it may be possible to help individuals, now much more motivated and with a higher level of self-image, to move to a new work lifestyle. Flynn *et al*. (1987) indicate that diagnostic category has little predictive value for subsequent job outcome and success. Other factors are important. It is clear from the work of Borgen, Amundson and Biela (1987) that physically disabled persons go through major periods of depression and apathy in relation to job placement. The authors observed oscillation in feelings over time. These oscillations were associated with accident and injury, efforts at accepting a disability condition, reaction to job search and failure, and adaptation to retraining procedures. Such reactions seem basic to many stress and unfamiliar processes, and are not restricted to one type of disability.

Similar effects are seen, for example, in the field of depression. Individuals often come to hospital, receive counselling and advice, but find that their major concerns continue. Sometimes individuals are provided with day hospital or other treatment, but are then sent back to the home backgrounds which were associated with the depression in the first place. Often individuals are given advice over finance, employment and personal issues which they are unable to take in. Again this is expected, given the model described. Verbal involvement, when it is possible, should be provided at a very basic level. Recent experiments dealing with verbal reinforcement of positive self-images seem to have some effect, but such training involves a very concrete level of vocabulary. Where visual and tactile aspects of environment are associated with depression it is unlikely that verbal input alone will overcome the difficulties. Other approaches are recommended. Although in such instances in the initial stages of breakdown, and in emergencies, verbal contact may be important, it is argued that tactile and visual involvement is likely to be essential. Both in the case of workers returning to their work environments after accidents, and in the case of psychiatric patients returning to their home environments, it is recommended that the change is initiated on a short-term basis, the individual is provided with a support worker who is familiar to the individual and can lend 'a practical hand' in the environment, essentially at a non-verbal level. Such involvement is likely to provide support and assistance which will enable the individual to survive in the environment. To the best of our knowledge, except at a very lay volunteer level or in cases of major physical hardship, such detailed psychological and social support is not regularly provided.

Impulsivity and the model

Meichenbaum (1971a) indicates that many cognitively impulsive children make a wide range of errors and have rapid decision times, but reflective children tend to make fewer errors and have a long decision time. In relation to the verbalization of these children he notes that private speech of impulsive children consisted of immature stimulatory content, whereas the reflective preschoolers used their private speech in a more mature, more instrumental self-guiding fashion. Kagan (1984) argues for a 'reflection impulsivity' domain which is related to children's academic and emotional behaviour. Some children appear interested in minimizing error and take considerable time to search for the best solution. Within the rehabilitation model it is argued that environmental stress will drive people from a more reflective stage towards impulsivity leading to greater error in problem-solving situations. Thus not only do we believe that language will move from the covert to the overt under stressful stimulation, it is also argued that language will move from goal-oriented behaviour to much more immature speech including spontaneous and imprecise answers involving considerable error. Indeed in the work of Norrie (1970) this was clearly demonstrated, for as individuals moved to tasks which were far too difficult for them they began to increase the range of irrelevant, non-task-oriented verbalization. Meichenbaum and Goodman (1969) also noted that impulsive children tend to show significantly less verbal control of inhibitory motor behaviour, and a greater magnitude of error, than reflective children on a Luria-type verbal control task. This again is consistent with the model that we are putting forward.

Meichenbaum has underlined the importance of self-instructional training for impulsive hyperactive children and recommends imagery manipulations. For us this is the equivalent of visual training. The importance of synthesizing and internalizing verbal information and modelling of that verbal information seems to be important. We argue that material which is at a visual level is more likely to become relevant to a person under stress, and therefore enhance learning because it enhances attention. On the other hand, the advantage of verbal performance is that it helps to generalize knowledge and application to a wider field, but it can only be success-fully employed when the individual is in a mode to deal with this wider area. The verbal behaviour can then enhance attention and direction in a wider range of tasks.

Thus the level and mode chosen for teaching or treatment depends on the level of functioning in the individual and the state of his development and stress.

Meichenbaum also talks about instructional ways of imaging methods of handling anxiety. In our model this represents one of the treatment modalities that might be used in such circumstances. In another study Meichenbaum (1971b) indicated the importance of modelling therapy in snake-phobic clients. Patients' fears were dealt with by instructing them to remain relaxed and calm through the use of slow and deep breathing. This is an interesting example because it is, in effect, encouraging individuals to start performing in a tactile and kinaesthetic mode. It implicitly involves using the regression model whereby individuals are enabled to perform successfully at a low level of behaviour, thus establishing a firm and effective base-line before attempting to bring behaviour up to a standard which can control normal situations. If we combine this visual self-imaging with actual external or overt signs of behaviour, such as using a method for visual training through videotape techniques (Dowrick and Biggs, 1983), much greater impact should be found. Indeed Dowrick (1978), working with a mother and child, used edited videotapes of the couple to show acceptable behaviour interaction, which resulted in dramatic improvement in performance.

The model and response uncertainty

In the field of memory, Mosley (1980) notes the major effects that unfamiliar stimuli have on mildly mentally handicapped persons resulting in poor performance. It is interesting that Mosley (1985) suggests that some of the uncertainty of responding, presumably in unfamiliar situations, is not a memory process as such, but response uncertainty. This agrees with previous findings cited by Brown and others, and again stresses the importance of the unfamiliarity dimensions in a wide range of practical situations. As Mosley states

In conclusion the revised model reveals that mildly retarded subjects fail to extract and/or hang on to the salient or relevant aspects of stimulus situations. And in turn [this] leads to poor performance in situations where unfamiliar or novel stimuli are employed and poor performance in situations where familiar stimuli are employed, but the information load is high.

Learned helplessness

Many of chronically mentally ill people suffer, in part, from learned helplessness (Abramson, Seligman & Teasdale, 1978; Seligman, 1979). This learned helplessness fits well with the model that has been put forward, for it suggests that individuals have been forced by the situation given to them to rely more and more on simpler modalities. The simple or initial modalities, such as tactile and visual, do not allow for long-term planning or the control of the environment by verbal means. Once again, however, the model argues that chronically mentally ill persons or individu who have been institutionalized for long periods of time cannot be removed rap to the community, but have to go through phases of programming in order to reach this point. If the model is accepted, curricular packages need to be developed to take into account each stage of development. Curricular packages that exist tend not to fit into a coherent theme of rehabilitation education. This type of planning recognizes that the rehabilitation process will be a long one.

Short- and long-term strategies

Many of the issues that we have dealt with in the model look to the development of continua and modalities which eventually bring about long-term strategy-building. Most of this, when applied by the client, is carried out at a conscious level and there is considerable work suggesting that once such plans are organized, then the activity is no longer thought through at a conscious level, but automated. Such long-term planning cannot be achieved overnight and requires gradual introduction, moving along the continua described, to a level where this can be done automatically.

Short-term strategies are seen in the area of delinquency and criminal behaviour. It has been pointed out by Coleman (1986) that many criminals, who have a long record of activity, may obtain funds through stealing but spend these funds very rapidly. After this period they are forced to return to the depressing reality that they have not got the wherewithal to sustain an effective form of lifestyle. This rapid use of the gains of crime links with the model in two ways: (1) concrete and immediate gratification occurs because the individuals are functioning at a concrete and overt level, and (2) their responses are not, on the whole, planned over a long period of time, but immediately, despite the fact this may lead to reconviction. Their behaviour is concrete both in terms of type of response and also in temporal terms. Coleman notes that the thief often speaks of an excitement associated with committing the offence. Yet the method of using what is stolen suggests emotional gratification is at a very simple or immature level. This has been linked to the early background of criminals and their behaviour.

More support for the application of the rehabilitation model can be assumed given the fact that these individuals are often from an adverse or unsatisfactory home background, which is lacking in structure and loving and supportive parental models (Belsen, 1975). If this is accepted, then the rehabilitation strategies for overcoming criminal behaviour lie in two fields: (1) in prevention, through the provision of appropriate early environments, an idea which is not new; and (2) once crimes have been committed, in rehabilitation by a gradual process of structured training; that is providing individuals with strategies to use development processes. Thus tactile and visual modalities should be accepted, and short- and long-term reward provided within the framework provided earlier. This will necessitate opportunities for exploration and application within the normal environment on a structured and controlled basis. Such an approach, which can be expected to take many years, is one which is foreign to the administration of penitentiary services. Once again, structure and control does not imply authoritarian direction, but the use of structured strategies which aim at internalizing those learning processes which will enhance both environment and self-control.

Conclusion

An attempt has been made to illustrate how models of rehabilitation, through one particular example, can provide opportunities for understanding and rethinking our approaches to a variety of disabling conditions. It is not that the facts are new but that the information can be put into a generic model from which ideas and processes for dealing with a wide range of behaviours can be derived. In some cases practice has provided examples, but they tend to be isolated and not linked to an overriding rationale for service delivery. This is unfortunate for it means that efficient, but limited, practice is not passed on to students as practitioners, thus resulting in a lack of generalization of knowledge.

CHAPTER EIGHT

Rehabilitation vignettes

Introduction

The following pages introduce a series of vignettes illustrating some common social and psychological problems. Some recommendations are provided and some leads to application of the arguments put forward in the previous chapters. It is hoped the reader will attempt to apply various details of the rehabilitation model and think of new examples. The use of the continua, both in terms of education and training and in terms of behavioural development often, in our experience, leads to a rethinking of particular issues.

Vignette 1

John is 15 years of age and comes from a poor socioeconomic background where there is some indication of child abuse. Recently he has suffered from epileptic seizures during the late evening. The rehabilitation educator wishes to teach John some mathematic skills and introduce problem-solving strategies.

There are a number of concerns in this particular situation. From an application of the model and general knowledge in the area, some statements can be made about John which should be verifiable from his records. These lead to suggestions on the type of approach which might be made.

There is some evidence that John comes from an adverse environment and that he is reaching an age where some cognitive acceleration might be expected. He is also, because of the type of home situation from which he comes, likely to show much lower verbal than non-verbal functioning ability. His epileptic seizures late in the day may be associated with fatigue and stress and therefore the introduction of learning materials in the evening hours are to be avoided. The sudden introduction of a problem-solving strategy is likely to cause new stress, and therefore unless it is gradually introduced with some considerable care it could increase the level of epileptic seizures. Furthermore, from the description provided it is likely that John is not functioning well within the verbal modality. It would therefore be wise to introduce problem-solving strategies at a visual and tactile level. Given the fact that he will be in a new situation, which will increase stress, it is suggested that the major principles of learning should be provided; that is, adaptation to unfamiliar situations, sessions of short duration and an accent on visual cues. Encouragement to externalize behaviour would be appropriate, but the use of highly encoded abstract vocabulary would probably do more harm than good. It would probably be important to cut down extraneous simulation. But all of this may be of little value unless something can be done with the much wider picture of treating the child abuse and general early experiences of low stimulation. Gaps in knowledge and emotional development are likely to have occurred, and these should be explored in relation to enhancing both emotional and cognitive stability through structured positive learning experiences. Some work (Sgroi, 1982) suggests that one of the most helpful ways of treating children who have been sexually abused is through the use of visual arts therapy. The method of self-expression also including play therapy, dance and drama (Warren, 1984) allows children to resolve the pain and trauma through the process of creating something that represents those feelings which is not in a verbal mode.

A comprehensive approach which involves the family and home situations may be critical. Without this, recovery and development may be restricted, and removal from the home development would have to be considered. A stable and structured environment is required along the lines suggested in the model. Rehabilitation will take a long time, and an increased amount of regression is likely to take place when intervention first occurs, thus leading to even lower performance levels. Such reduced performance or age-inappropriate behaviour must be explained to the parents, so that they refrain from reacting too intensely and causing increased stress.

Vignette 2

Michael, who is 10 years old, attends an elementary school. He has been to three other schools and reports indicate a series of problems and failures. His reading attainment is that of an average 6-year-old. His WISC test shows Verbal IQ of 69 and Performance IQ of 85. His mother says teachers do not understand him and do not know how to teach. She knows 'because she has read the latest books'. She indicates that she expects an IPP to be developed and wishes to meet with teachers to discuss teaching that she is doing at home.

Michael, like John, shows a range of developmental problems and although he may not come from an adverse environment, for he appears to have a very supportive mother, nevertheless he may be under stress at home in teaching situations provided by his mother. Further, he has attended a range of schools which suggest that he will have been taught by different methods at different times, a problem which is often overlooked by teaching personnel. Thus this aspect of environment is variable and does not meet the requirements of early structure. The introduction to basic reading and mathematics may have been inconsistent, defeating the learning processes which are clearly described earlier. It is obviously important in this case to introduce and establish a structured background and to ensure that early learning processes have been dealt with effectively. Regression is expected, thus earlier levels of learning, for example pre- and primary-reading skills, must be introduced. Daily routines involving brief time periods and small but frequent amounts of new material are likely to be valuable. How frequent and how small can only be gauged by

e and practical assessment procedures, the results of which should
ition of the teaching situation. It is also important to ensure that
with education is reduced, so one of the first aims may be to ask
out of the teaching and deal with the parenting processes.

r individual programme planning is, of course, a sensible one, and
se days recognize, because they have read a large amount of the
literature, that this approach is important. It is the sort of issue which can also be
used as a confrontational tactic with schools! An Individual Programme Planning
process should be undertaken and an explanation given of the types of performance
problems that Michael will be facing. Again the discrepancy between lower verbal,
compared with performance, intelligence, raises the question of how the teacher can
anticipate which teaching strategies will best match John's learning style. However,
what is readily apparent is that the basics of structure have not been developed in
the verbal area. Utilization of visual and tactile components in learning strategies
is important. Verbal instruction should be simple and employed at first as a support
to visual demonstration.

Vignette 3

*Joan, aged 22, attends a vocational training agency. She has an IQ of 65 Verbal
and 80 Performance on the WAIS. She has poor self-concept and makes little
progress. Her parents say she is handicapped and cannot be expected to learn. They
wish the agency to look after her during the day and they will take care of her on
nights and weekends. They say 'Please do not bother us with meetings'.*

This particular case raises a number of important issues. The relatively low verbal
intelligence level suggests the individual comes from a somewhat restricted environment and/or that organic factors are present. There is a need in building programme
models to provide practical, visual and tactile stimulation. However, there is also
ample evidence that the individual may have very poor self-image and be in a
position where she has become dependent on others for her responses and activities.
Learned helplessness is a possibility. Motivation would seem low, and it is apparent
that the parents do not provide a very positive environment for optimism in learning
new behaviour.

In such situations it is very important to shift the attitude of parents by engaging
the parents in reframing family activities in their own setting, to support growth
informally rather than in artificial agency environments. It is important to demonstrate in very practical, social, non-verbal situations that the individual can attain
some goals, which are of practical use, not only to the individual, but also within
the family context, thus increasing Joan's ability to control some of her own environment, while reducing the amount of responsibility of the parents and freeing up their
time. However, this is not going to be achieved by verbal counselling alone; nor is
it going to be done by relatively advanced levels of education. The requirement is
for very simple, short-term, highly structured tasks with individuals who will help
Joan to develop a high level of self-respect for more successful performance.
Rehabilitation needs may occur over a long period, but each new stage of learning

may involve a relatively short but intense period of structured teaching. To do this comprehensively over time, functional current baseline assessment is critical.

Vignette 4

Mr and Mrs Jones have a new baby who has been diagnosed as having Down's syndrome. They come to an agency for advice, believing the agency has knowledgeable people who can inform and help. There will be a number of issues that are likely to arise, and these concerns have to be dealt with by the parents.

In this particular case the model is being applied not to the individual who has Down's syndrome, but the parents. At the time of delivery of a handicapped child it is known that a number of reactions and concerns frequently arise (Wolfensberger, 1967; Younghusband *et al.*, 1970; Byrne and Cunningham, 1985) and these fit well with the model of behaviour that has been described. Regression in parental behaviour may occur. There may be guilt, anger, fear and anxiety. Certainly a very high level of emotional responding is anticipated, whether this is made overtly or covertly. Indeed, the model anticipates that much of the emotional behaviour will take place at an overt level, particularly in the home environment. The regression of behaviour will possibly reach tactile, visual and concrete verbal levels. The nature of the problem is such that parents are unlikely to be able to comprehend easily what is said to them at a verbal level by a counsellor or therapist. They are likely to require visual and tactile input which will enable them to stabilize an effective baseline and develop an understanding of the facts presented. Their non-verbal behaviour is likely to regress and a high level of error is likely to occur. This is why contact with other parents, people who have been through a similar process, is probably an important method of providing information and experience. This provides for modelling, emotional support and visual, if not tactile, contact which is consistent with previous arguments. Although the process may not be a long one, it should be recognized that emotional responses are appropriate and should be accepted. Gradually responses will be internalized and more elaborate and supportive responses will come forward with periods of natural regression when the parents move into new unfamiliar stages of life with their child (i.e. toilet training, starting preschool programmes, entering the education system, etc.). The need to observe other parents in action who have similar problems is important as stressors emerge. When verbal counselling is requested, it should be done with visual aids and include opportunities for repetition, as knowledge at a verbal level is likely to be distorted or forgotten. Again the opportunity to do this in a familiar environment with the counsellor seeing the child is relevant, not only because advice can be more practical and supports can be more effective, but because the visual and tactile involvement are necessary. Positive responses to the child from the advisor are critical. It is of interest in this context that Cunningham and Sloper (1977) work suggests the involvement of a health visitor (e.g. public health nurse) to the home is one of the most supportive aspects of involvement for the parents of young Down's syndrome children.

Vignette 5

John suffers from cerebral palsy and is 10 years of age. He has a right hemiplegia.
He has difficulty in playing with many toys, particularly with items such as Lego
blocks. He cannot put them together to form recognizable shapes involving ten items
and three colours, as his same-age peers may do, to create an interesting play
activity. He travels a long distance to special school each day.

John will have many other specific problems, particularly those involving space
and motor skills, but probably also difficulties in the verbal area. Yet where verbal
development has taken place this may be used as an effective crutch and support in
carrying out non-verbal tasks. Overt verbalization from the child, using his own
words, may be effective in such situations. The need to cut down stress will be
important because stress will effect motor movement, making early learning more
difficult. For example, many such children are transported by bus to schools where
it is thought the environment may be more supportive. Yet bus transportation is
known to cause fatigue, and amongst many children aggression is increased. In this
case it is likely that the fatigue from transportation will make early learning much
more difficult. Any form of stress must be reduced to a minimum if effective learning structures are to be provided. Learning practical domestic skills in a home
environment is extremely important, and wherever possible the access to the local
community resources to practise cognitive skills is necessary, not only to teach
transfer, but to maintain motivation. Quick success will also be important, as reward
normally comes slowly to such children. The model suggests a high level of structure and organization with an accent on familiarity. Concrete visual performance,
with possible auditory supports, may be critical. Size and weight of toys, small
changes in unit size towards normality and the opportunity to verbalize, along with
small time periods for practice, and the reduction of extraneous stimulation, may
all be relevant in teaching manipulation of toys. However, such children require
social stimulation at other times so that they keep active and involved. The danger
is that deprivation of social interaction, because of impairment, may worsen self-
concept and motivation for learning. However, it is not just a matter of reduced
stimulation overall, but looking at stimulation at crucial points in time, particularly
in early learning situations and in certain stages of emotional development.

Vignette 6

Gillian is going to her first job interview. She has a Verbal IQ of 69 and Performance
IQ of 85. She has been in a vocational training agency for 3 years and is now
believed to be ready for a work environment.

This type of situation can be expected to provide a number of interesting and
challenging problems. First of all, Gillian's language level is lower than her non-
verbal skills, therefore it is likely that she can perform at a much higher level in
semi-skilled and skilled work than people recognize, provided the verbal component
is reasonably low. However, when people go for interviews they are involved in
verbal communication and therefore unlikely to do well under these circumstances.

Staff should provide her with opportunities to practise interviewing procedures before she goes to the critical job interview. It is also important that her potential employers know of the likely relationship between non-verbal and verbal functioning. It should also be recognized that an individual who has been in a vocational training agency, particularly if social and home living skill and community training have not been involved, will show considerable behavioural regression when the individual commences employment. The individual's level of performance will diminish at first, recovering as adaptation to the work situation takes place. Of course, as indicated from the model, it should be possible to deal with transfer and generalization, at least in part, during the earlier training process. However, unfortunately this is not often done.

It should be recognized that she may not effectively recall what is said by others in interviewing situations, although she will remember quite well what she has personally said. Attempts should be made to simulate interviews for her, giving practical examples of questions, tone of voice, seating arrangements, etc. As far as possible the work situation should also be simulated. The amount of standing, sitting and work pressure are all important variables, along with type of lighting and noise. The recommendations for how training is carried out in these circumstances are implicit in the model provided. It is important to keep other activities and experiences unchanged during this period, and this particularly applies to her support worker or job trainer, who should be a familiar person. Consistent, familiar external structure will become very important during the initial placement period.

Vignette 7

George is a 27-year-old engineer who has been in a car accident and was in a coma for 6 months. He gradually regains use of gross hand movements, and some fine movements in his right hand. He has some language problems including aphasia. He is sent home and has some difficulties in making his needs known. George is married, but has no children.

Individuals who are moved back to home from a hospital situation are likely to show very considerable regression when first confronted with what was a familiar environment. It is now unfamiliar, because many of the things that they could do previously can no longer be tackled, bringing frustration and stress. Feelings of anxiety and ineffectiveness follow, self-image declines, and external structure needs to be increased.

George's wife must be informed about the behavioural effects that are likely to occur. In our experience this is rarely done. Regression is likely to be sudden and cause George extra difficulties. He, too, must know about the effects of changing his environment. Gradually, provided the regression is not too great and he has some insight into the process, he will begin to adapt to situations. But there will be a tendency to over-protect him and not let him employ skills, because people do not recognize the abilities and attainments which still exist. People will respond to his verbal responses rather than non-verbal aspects of performance. For example, the authors have been in a situation where an individual was able to plan a patio, even though he was suffering from major problems of aphasia. Medical and non-medical staff, and the client's wife, had assumed the individual could not succeed. However, demonstration of ability to do this task indicated not only to the client and his wife, but also to professional practitioners, that he had effective skills at his command.

Capitalization on existing resources is critical, but cannot be done unless there are practical baseline assessments. Structure is necessary, but this can be gradually removed. Short term intervals, possibly tactile and visual involvement will be critical, and speed of response may be extremely slow. It must be recognized that the rehabilitation process will be a long one; therefore rapid gains, particularly in new learning, may not be as quick as the individual would hope. Further cyclical responding will occur, frustrating the participant and his supporters. This must be taken into account with structure being increased and decreased as required. The involvement of persons skilled in providing this type of flexibility is important. Opportunities to transfer skills are also invaluable.

Vignette 8

Jane has suffered from a depressive illness with suicidal tendencies. She has been sent to a day hospital after spending 3 weeks within a psychiatric ward of a general hospital. During this period she goes home in the evenings and returns to the day hospital each morning, where she carries out basket weaving and macramé. She shows considerable frustration with the tasks in the day hospital and is seen by some to be an irritable patient. She has recently gone through a divorce and there is nobody else living at home.

There has been a recognition for some time that day services and a more social approach to mental ill health are necessary. Some, (Jones, 1968; Bierer and Evans, 1969), have recognized and developed centres for the application of social psychiatry. Although these are important steps to the development of community-oriented services, we argue that it is also important to get away from meaningless activities in artificial environments that have controls which are not necessarily useful for the individual. Without the delivery of supports to the home and immediate local community the rehabilitation process is likely in many instances to be ineffective, and to delay the recovery process.

In this vignette return to the home environment is likely to precipitate further regression and depression, leaving the person feeling unable to cope with the complexity of the life situation. Self-image is very poor, and lack of ability to function within the home environment will further reinforce this image. The very fact that the individual cannot see the relevance of the occupational therapy, and her anger at the situation, compound the problem. In her situation no professional person has visited the home to see the condition it is in, nor have they calculated the various supports which are required. Yet this is vital if Jane is to be helped. Home help must not be directed towards doing everything, but rather allowing and encouraging the individual to organize his or her priorities at a very simple and practical level in order gradually to take over control in running the home with success. This can lead to improvement in self-image. The person who supports in the home must therefore have a very considerable knowledge of behavioural structure, and the model provides for a number of ways in which help can be given in this direction. Obviously structure and long-term planning are necessary. Structure means the setting of short-term goals, at visual and concrete levels (for example, a simple timetable or chart of proposed activities). Tactile support and comfort will be necessary. Regression will frequently occur, and support may be necessary at particular points during the day. This will include periods where the individual must be allowed to regress, including periods for sleep. Such behaviour follows personal idiosyncrasies and can only be catered for if there is a highly individualized programme. It should be recognized that many of the behaviours the individual shows will be because of regression, and the operational level will tend to be tactile, visual and concrete verbal. The individual will very often seem preoccupied and not respond to verbal requests. Occupation in the tactile area should be with items with which they formerly had some interest, not with new items for which they do not see relevance, and often require new or original learning, a requirement which, according to the model, will do more harm than good because of the stress involved.

Areas involving more abstract thought will need support or have to be taken over by a responsible advocate. For example, in another case where the individual, during periods of manic depression, was spending vast sums of money, it would have been helpful if a guardian had been appointed to look after financial issues. Regression effects mean that for short periods the individual lacked competence in dealing with such abstract and verbal matters. An effective guardian will vary the amount of controls in place over time. It is important to recognize that the individual cannot deal with abstract and long-term processes at particular points in time. The new Dependent Adults's Acts, in Australia and Canada, demonstrate some of the protection that can be provided through legislation that recognizes changing levels of competence in decision-making in an individual over time. Unfortunately the legal and health professions have not fully developed the type of sensitive structures required to deal with such regressive yet fluid situations.

Vignette 9

James suffered an accident at work which involved a major back injury. He has been off work for some months and cannot return to the physical type of activity that was previously required in his work. He has received advice from a variety of sources but is not making positive adaptation, and has not yet chosen a new field of employment.

Very often such cases are a major challenge because the individual is dealing with considerable pain which lowers level of performance. It also reduces the amount of time that can be spent on particular activities. Stress and, therefore, the types of behaviours that result, including depression and irritability, are likely to affect close personal relationships. Furthermore the individual recognizes he cannot go back to his previous employment, and it is quite likely that a more sedentary job involving verbal components is suggested. This represents an area in which the individual was not functioning well in the first place. Very often such situations give rise to major difficulties and require retraining. Yet training involves new learning, which itself tends to result in further stress and regression in behaviour. This confirms the individual's perception of disability and decreases motivation to participate. In such situations it is important that, through visual demonstration and visual aspects of counselling, the individual sees what has happened to other individuals. One way of doing this is through videotape. The individual family members must recognize the long-term goals involved and recovery may have to be directed through non-vocational means. This involves a training programme which can result in greater command of a familiar environment. Such an approach has profound implications for financial support and compensatory financial allowances to such individuals. We see the importance of adaptation to the community and home and the development of leisure time skills. Here the individual can gain control of environmental aspects that will raise self-image and motivation and, thereby, cognitive problem-solving ability. It then becomes possible to move to adaptation in a new job situation. Obviously, if a suitable job is available with close approximation to skills in the previous job such a strategy may be unnecessary. However in our experience this is frequently not the case.

In this particular instance another issue arises: the psychological control of pain. Although much advice may be given around technical aspects of pain control, such as drugs, behavioural strategies to deal with pain are not often discussed with the individual and the family. Behaviour will follow the model. It will become more overt and language will regress, tactile and visual components will predominate in the situation and, as a result, the individual will not function in his or her customary way. Attempts to regain previous levels of performance will result in further pain, thus increasing the difficulties and the chances of failure, with consequent loss of self-image. In this particular situation simple strategies to deal with pain as a learning phenomenon are important. The individual must be given insight into the need for slowness in behaviour, must be shown that small but frequent periods of activity during the day may be desirable, and that regressive behaviour, in terms of overt performance and expression of pain, are to be expected and are not abnormal. Indeed, such regression may be a means of adapting as a first step in obtaining a baseline or consolidation of behaviour from which gains can later be made. Progress will be slow, with an immense amount of variability, including oscillation of behaviour levels which are demotivating in their own right. A knowledge of these processes, both by the family and the individual, is important to an understanding about growth and the re-establishment of an acceptable baseline of performance. Visual indications (e.g. photograph albums, videotapes) of progress, however slow, are important for both James and his family. Tactile responses from loved ones and friends and professionals are desirable. Motor behaviour may be gross to begin with, thus accidents (e.g. breaking things, falling and burns) are more likely to occur in the home. Awareness of such possibilities is important, but opportunities to try things out are equally necessary. Otherwise the environment becomes depriving and opportunities for recovery are reduced. In such instances prosthetic devices may play an important role but their introduction may be accompanied by regression behaviour associated with unfamiliarity and stress. Often resistance to using such aids may have to be dealt with in a supportive manner that tolerates many trials before James adapts and accepts the value of such aids for his unique circumstances.

Summary

This chapter has attempted to give examples of the relevance of various facets of the model which deals with features of learning and performance and environment to a variety of disabling conditions. It is recognized the model is merely one way of organizing information, and can only act as a guideline. Over-involvement in the model could prevent professionals from recognizing other possible approaches. Yet at this stage in practice, the concepts provided through the model provoke questions and suggest strategies which may be tested. An account has been given of the various practical possibilities which arise from a consideration of the model with evidence from different areas of disability and disorder. Together they illustrate the relevancy of the model to intervention practices. By supplying a number of simple vignettes, examples have been given of practical application within the field of rehabilitation.

In summary, it is important to recognize that effective baseline assessment and individual programme planning is employed. Various facets of the model can be used as a guide. Indeed one use of the model is to give practitioners a general format and language structure which can provide a framework for the development and exchange of practical ideas.

CHAPTER NINE

Relevance of the model to service delivery systems

Introduction

This chapter is not intended to be a comprehensive survey of management and administrative techniques, but a look at the model of rehabilitation and its possible application within the field of management and administration. In the field of management, relatively little work has been done in terms of the application of behavioural systems to management processes within the health and social fields, and certainly the application of rehabilitation techniques and models to the field of management is almost non-existent. Within the range of management material that is available many recommendations are made for the development and proper administration of management systems. Such books not only provide advice and comment, but provide a range of techniques and assessment devices to evaluate management processes (Schulberg and Baker, 1979; Shaw, 1984). Although many have been concerned to look at the lifestyle and employment satisfaction of employees (Mendaglio and Swanson, 1986), the effect of changing management models or systems is rarely examined in relation to treatment or recovery rates of clients. Indeed in the behavioural realm the rehabilitation process, regardless of disability, has taken a back seat in terms of its relevance to the development of management processes and structures.

An integrated approach

The rehabilitation model we have discussed suggests a range of recommendations which might be appropriate for meeting the needs of specific clients within the rehabilitation field. First of all, it has been argued that any rehabilitation model must be a comprehensive process. That is, it must look at all systems relating to the individual's functioning and in many cases will be required to provide rehabilitative techniques to deal with vocational, social, leisure time and home living aspects of lifestyle. Each area must be represented by a continuum of training components as described earlier. In current practice this is only partially recognized, in that different agencies or different parts of agencies deal with the process of training, often as a care function.

But just as the client is subjected to possible regression effects under stress and difficulty, so is the agency and its staff. Thus we suggest that the model provided earlier applies not just to the client, but also the various persons who serve the client. In building and changing service systems we should examine the possible behavioural effects which may assist or harm the client.

Agency philosophy

Most rehabilitation agencies provide care during vocational maintenance, or care in relation to home residence. Such are rudimentary support systems and in terms of our model represent concrete rather than abstract notions of rehabilitation. Such services are typified by the following characteristics:

1. they have physical plants,
2. they are generally in non integrated areas of the community,
3. they are generally of large size,
4. they have ill-defined philosophies,
5. they have hierarchical management structures,
6. a large number of clients do not show major and positive changes,
7. placement rates are low.

Our concern is that at present few people are being rehabilitated out of agencies into the community, partly because of lack of availability of jobs, but also because of the lack of integration of training programmes. Unless there is a comprehensive philosophy that is developed between the different wings or areas of a programme, it is unlikely that effective rehabilitation will take place. Effective philosophy suggests not only must different agencies work closely together, but that it might be better if a comprehensive agency system were developed to provide a coherent rehabilitation approach. The evidence that is available in the field, whether from the field of physical disability or from mental handicap, whether it is in learning disabilities or in emotional disturbances, suggests that, for the most part, individuals are not handicapped in one but in several domains. Therefore just in the same way as client deficits exist, and in the same way that different and varied needs arise, so programme delivery needs to be comprehensive and integrated. It should be recognized that the same developmental and rehabilitation needs exist in each domain and the domains are interdependent. It is incumbent on any management team to ensure that staff working in one area of client rehabilitation are knowledgeable about other areas of the individual's rehabilitation.

If different agencies are involved in the process of rehabilitation then it is important that agencies do not get together or work together simply because it is convenient for geographical, or financial or space reasons, but because they have similar philosophies and goals.

Some recommendations follow, and can be viewed as relevent to an agency with many programmes, or to different agencies which combine their efforts to provide comprehensive service.

An integrated philosophy

Any agency which offers services in more than one domain for an individual should ensure that its staff from the various service areas share an integrated and consistent philosophy. All staff must understand the major goals and aims of the programme. The goals should be maintained throughout the agency. For example, individuals who are placed in a unit for vocational training should not find in the home living area that they are abandoned to simple care, or that staff in the second unit hold different goals in mind compared with their vocational colleagues. It is totally unacceptable to have a philosophy of care and protection in one unit, where individuals are not viewed as rehabilitatable, and a philosophy of normalization in another unit which works with the same individuals. In our experience such contradictions are common. When such primary differences occur, a full examination of staff and agency philosophy is necessary.

Agency and client goals

Devices such as the Marlett and Hughson Programme Priorities Scale (1977), now exist in the field for examining agency philosophical and programme constructs, and needs assessment models are common in many educational areas (English and Kaufman, 1975). Very often agencies at board or advisory level, or government departments, have certain beliefs which reflect their philosophy and goals. The philosophy and goals of middle management and front-line staff may be very different. It is essential to clarify and agree on these goals, which should be publicly stated.

Behavioural treatment is aimed at meeting very personal goals and general statements are inadequate. If potential staff do not hold priorities consistent with the goals of the agency they should not be employed. If the society membership or community of potential rehabilitees does not agree with or accept the agency goals, then a very serious situation exists which should be subject to critical evaluation and modification. This view is consistent with an advocacy model where the individual client's motivation and interests must be viewed as part of the rehabilitation process. In a medical model the individual is traditionally seen as a person who receives services and has processes applied to him. Rehabilitation education assumes the individuals are an organic part of the service, and what happens with them is dependent on each individual's conscious support and involvement.

This view recognizes some of the important conceptual changes taking place in community service. It provides for a model which places the client at the centre of decision-making. It accepts that rehabilitation cannot effectively occur unless conscious involvement and practial participation comes from the client. Thus a partnership is formed. This is consistent with the aims of the rehabilitation model described earlier, for effective rehabilitation must involve the improvement of self-image, a reduction of stress and the involvement of familiar persons. The better the support system and blending with client concerns, the more likely it is that rehabilitation can advance to a phase where higher-level verbal strategies can be employed. But, as indicated elsewhere, behaviour to begin with is often less well developed and considerable regression has taken place. Thus non-verbal or low verbal strategies occur. Overt language and visual and tactile responsiveness are important, but cognitive adaptation requires learning and internalization or automization of rehabilitation processes. To achieve this, the individual must be personally and actively involved.

In the instances of a very low level of personal client involvement, individuals acceptable to the client must take over this role—parents, spouses, close friends—but rarely professional personnel—at least in the first instance. Thus close relatives form a major part in the rehabilitation bridging process. By a process of 'bonding', modelling, encouragement and continuous involvement they may enable the low-functioning individual to eventually identify with the rehabilitation process, making it more speedy and effective. This rarely takes place in the traditional medical model, which often does things to individuals, generally without their understanding and frequently without their conscious involvement. There is little internalization of the strategy or process though the individual may do what he or she is told.

Client numbers and management

In most rehabilitation settings directors are remote from clients, either because there are so many clients or because there is a hierarchical system which removes the director, both in time and space, from the delivery of the front-line service. Many agencies have separate directors or managers for residential programmes and separate managers for vocational or social programmes. This gives rise to a problem not only of coherency of philosophy, but of lack of a sense of 'programming-belong-ing' and direction for clients who are receiving, and personnel who are delivering, the service. In rehabilitation the accent is on client action and client learning. The client is never a bystander in the process while 'things' are done to him or her.

It is necessary to ensure a process of identification between the client and his or her programme, and this can best be done if the programme is client-centred and, where possible, client-activated. Otherwise (further) loss to self-image and motivation tends to occur.

Lateral versus vertical management structure

One of the problems is that there is frequently a hierarchical system whereby front-line staff in an agency report to middle management and so on, upward to the director or manager of the rehabilitation system. This executive officer in turn reports to an advisory or policy committee, sometimes in the form of an executive or board of directors (Kennett, 1986) (see Figure 14). Although there is at times a concept of team treatment or rehabilitation, professions generally maintain themselves in separate units, although working in departments or visiting another centre on occasion for therapeutic or assessment purposes. In some modern agencies a lattice model of responsibility is provided, with individuals relating to their professional department and their transdisciplinary programme (see Figure 15).

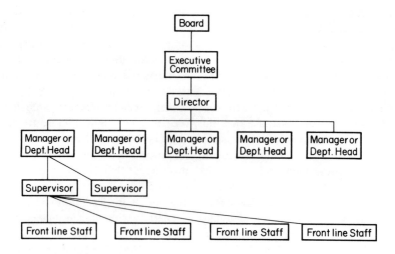

Figure 14. Traditional organization model.

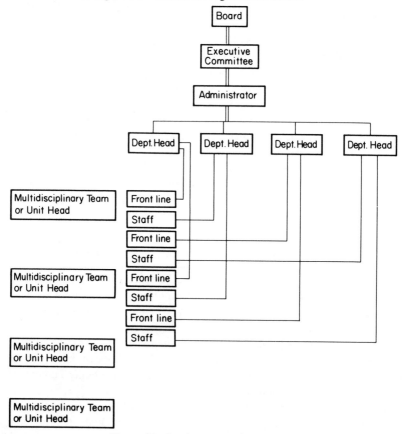

Figure 15. Lattice or matrix model.

One effective way to deal with some of these problems is to use a model of management whereby a director or manager of a programme is responsible for few clients, but these clients have their total programme integrated under the one system. Thus the director or manager becomes the person ultimately responsible for the philosophy and programme in home living, social, vocational, community, education and leisure areas. It is to this person that other staff relate. In Figure 16 the upper model shows each director partially responsible for nine clients, while in the lower model each director is entirely responsible for three different clients. Thus no new staffing costs are envisaged and the total number of clients served remains the same. It is suggested that such a unit should not be more than 50 clients in size, preferably fewer. Above this size directors or managers cannot know the clients intimately. The programme becomes depersonalized.

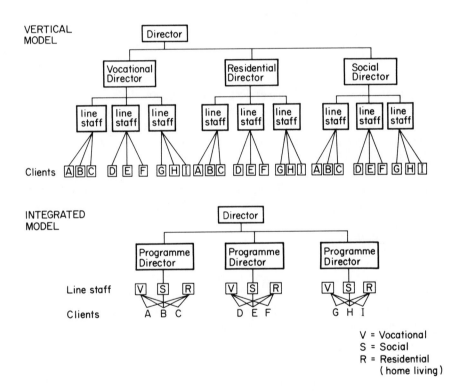

Figure 16. Examples of vertical and integrated models of management. Note that models have the same number of staff and clients.

One aspect of rehabilitation which seems to be of paramount importance is the recovery of self-image and motivation frequently lacking in individuals suffering trauma, and sometimes low or absent in individuals disabled from birth. This recovery or stabilization of adequate self-image or motivation is unlikely to occur when different professionals use different systems and different models, or have different goals for the client. The model proposed here requires that front-line staff, who are the ones administering the daily and integrated programme for the individual, have a major say in the development of programmes and philosophy for that individual. Obviously, as indicated earlier, if their views are foreign to the concept of rehabilitation they should not be employed within such a unit. However, given that their major concerns are directed towards the client, and they are sufficiently well trained, they should become organizers in the development of programme philosophy. Such programme philosophy should not simply be passed on from a central authority, but rather be developed by the programme team. The central authority is the 'servant' of front-line staff providing the wherewithal to develop and integrate individual programmes. The above leads not only to a different management structure, but also a new type of front-line worker.

In the field of medicine, once a hospital has decided to provide a heart transplant the team dealing with the particular situation has a leader who takes the organizing role in the operative procedures. We argue that the same type of ground-level organization and command must occur within the behavioural domain. Otherwise we find merely administrative and group structures being provided for the individual. For example, one of the major social services relates to financial allowances paid to, and provided for, individuals who have suffered from disability or handicap. This is often standard and limited in time (e.g. Worker's Compensation). This should not be based on a certain number of weeks for rehabilitation, but must recognize the highly diverse and variable rates of rehabilitation that occur. Rehabilitation is not a linear process but one with growth, plateaus, decrements and renewed growth in a variety of physical, social and behavioural dimensions. A financial and economic system must take these individualized patterns into account.

Communication systems

In order to develop effective rehabilitation strategies suitable communication systems must be developed. We have already seen within the rehabilitation model that communication systems are often non-verbal, and under stress even verbal systems move from abstract to more concrete modes of expression. This implies a number of moves within a management structure.

1. Directors of programmes must know the detail of their clients' cases and must be familiar with the individuals concerned.
2. They must be in direct and personal contact with their front-line staff.
3. Stresses can be caused by a variety of events related to crisis, or to the care system itself. This may occur amongst staff or clients. In such instances face-to-face contact is essential.
4. Management personnel, as well as other staff, must have skills in counselling.
5. The processes of motivation and self-image noted in relation to clients also occur in staff. Directors must promote a recognition of the causes, identification and treatment of stress and burnout (Mendaglio, 1982; Mendaglio and Swanson, 1986).

Many agencies distant from major hospitals are seen as auxiliary units, or as the Cinderella group associated with social welfare or health departments. Many rehabilitation units are still essentially perceived as care units for the most disabled clients. They have a low profile in the community and in the eyes of treatment and professional personnel in central services. A high profile for such centres and services must be developed if rehabilitation rates are to be enhanced.

Stress and burn-out

Part of the issue relates to self-image and attitudes amongst staff. Their self-image must be positive and protected. In recent years there has been considerable amount of discussion about the importance of stress and burn-out amongst staff (Mendaglio and Swanson, 1986), and this is readily recognized in organizations which are concerned with the training of persons who are likely to show major stress reactions. Stress in the rehabilitation areas falls under a number of headings:

1. Some individuals who require rehabilitation progress very slowly within the rehabilitation process. A recent study (Brown, Bayer and MacFarlane, 1985) undertaken in Canada suggests that many developmentally handicapped people may be 10 years or more within a particular rehabilitation agency. Their rates of progress may be slow or, perhaps because of the nature of the organizations involved, almost non-existent. In some cases deterioration is observed. Under such circumstances staff find it very hard to perceive themselves more than caretakers, and come to recognize the individual as incapable of improvement and development. This is a cause of stress to staff, client and family.

   The institution of refined assessment procedures which measure minor changes in performance is helpful not only in indicating methods to improve programme, but as a means of illustrating to staff and client that progress does occur. The motivating effects of this on clients and staff can be considerable. For example in the development of a pre-vocational study for severely mentally handicapped adults, Hughson, Berrien and Brown (1978) were confronted by statements from staff indicating that programming was a waste of time. Regular presentations by the unit's research assistant on individual progress in programme areas changed staff attitudes and helped to provide high motivation in the unit. Indeed the use of behavioural research assistants in such areas, to provide information feedback, is critical. Evans, Porterfield and Blunden (1986), and Blunden and Evans (1984) in their research, provide other examples of feedback and collaboration between various staff and allied groups in terms of evaluation of progress.

2. Individuals who have undergone a traumatic accident may be well aware of their previous capabilities and show a considerable degree of frustration, which manifests itself as aberrant, aggressive or depressive behaviour. Staff find such behaviour particularly difficult when it may take the form of either personally aggressive or antisocial behaviour. The involvement of consultants in behavioural management helps to alleviate such difficulties but, consistent with our

earlier arguments, this is not simply verbal advice but visual and 'hands-on' demonstration (Hughson, 1984).

3. Residential or home living staff who work in group homes may find training particularly stressful because of the time of day they are expected to function, and the content of the programme they are expected to deliver. Frequently the hours are long and often cover 'fatigue time'. Clients are often tired at the end of the day. The training or care period may involve weekend or vacations, which is stress time, because the programme is often highly unstructured at such periods. Some of the staff comments received in a research study by Beck-Ford et al. (1984) illustrate the problems. It is in these circumstances that the direct availability of a senior manager to interpret philosophy to staff is critical so that the development of a 'mission' is possible (Neufeldt, 1986). Both Marlett (1986) and Neufeldt, in this context, argue for the development of programme 'mythologies', that is concepts concerning aims and mission (Shaw, 1984) which become to be perceived as achievable, even though local attitudes may regard them as impossibilities. Such developments are critical if rehabilitation is to attain new and higher levels of success. Once again the function is largely a non-verbal one, involving essentially non-cognitive belief systems. Such beliefs are important to clients and can result in success, although they must be founded in reality. Feelings of optimism, challenge and hoped-for success are critical to both the client and the rehabilitation team.

4. In addition to the above major stressors there are other reasons for stress and burn-out. These have been stated clearly by a number of authors (Mendaglio and Swanson, 1986) in terms of signs or symptoms, such as staff feeling that they alone can work effectively because others are ineffective, that they must work long hours because they alone are responsible for an individual's programme, or that the management is uncaring. In other cases vague symptoms of a physical nature seem to be involved. Much of this may arise through lack of appropriate support and communication models in the system, or a lack of coherent philosophy so that people do not work as a team. Remoteness of the organization from central government or some similar control structure, inadequate leadership, etc., can also be relevant. Obviously a caring system, particularly a rehabilitation one, should pay attention to some of these concerns. The model of behavioural regression, structure and control also applies in these situations.

Dealing with stress

A number of possibilities have already been discussed for improving the situation of stress and burn-out. When staff show stress and regress in behaviour it would seem likely that their clients would show less improvement and development. That clients have concerns about such matters is apparent from a recent study by Brown et al. (1985), where clients' worries appear to be stated in terms of aggressive or negative comments from supervisors in training units.

It must also be borne in mind that staff are very poor at predicting which clients will improve, or will not improve, in behavioural and social terms. In other words it is essential that staff do not make long-term predictions about the success or otherwise of clients or come to believe which clients can carry out activity successfully or unsuccessfully. Such views or predictions tend to be underestimates, and are particularly negative when staff are under severe stress. Although prediction may be poor, clarity of programme goals, a stepwise approach to training, and a management system which supports the client and worker to have personal control in individual programming go some way to dealing with these issues.

It also appears that programmes which enjoy a feeling that their leadership conveys a sense of progress, innovation and development, foster staff who become even more enthusiastic, and pull together as a team. Staff burn-out tends to be low. It would also appear that under such circumstances success rates are likely to be at a higher level amongst clientele.

Familiar staff

There are already considerable data suggesting that nurturant and familiar models improve the recovery rates of clients. It also follows from this that clients should know their staff workers well. Although we hesitate to suggest that bonding takes place between staff and client, it is suggested that staff and client adapt to one another and can come to work as a team. The client who has a key worker throughout the rehabilitation process, including the follow-up process, is more likely to do well. Staff members are also likely to feel more effective since they see the results of their involvement. In addition to this conjoint familiarity, the concern to develop a team, and the development of integrated programming, leads to an atmosphere in which an effective individual rehabilitation plan can be constructed.

Individual programme plan and management

In the field of education in the United States, under Public Law 94-142, it has become mandatory that all children receive education regardless of handicap. From this model has developed the concept of an individual educational plan which, for the most part, has been incorporated in North America into individualized programme plans for most clients (Bernstein *et al.*, 1981). However, such planning does not always involve persons who are familiar with, or who have a large degree of contact with, the client. Marlett (1986) has argued that the system can develop into a bureaucratic approach which is of little value to the client.

The model described overcomes some of these difficulties, so that the individual programme plan or individual rehabilitation plan becomes an important part of the process of personal management and development. The individual rehabilitation plan involves key staff who work with the client. Such a plan involves meetings called by the chairperson of the group, who co-ordinates the programme and sees that the prescribed training is carried out. Wherever possible the client, plus parent or partner, advocate or next of kin, are involved in developing this plan, which is written with specific goals and strategies for achieving the goals. Timelines are provided as a guide. Such plans should be specific and fit well with the structured model provided earlier, but it should be recognized that, with progress, the goals and programme may become more abstract and include a range of transfer skills. Such a system needs to be worked out for every client. Given the type of model discussed in earlier chapters, it is essential that an appropriate assessment system is employed and information regularly recorded in a formal manner, enabling the development of a comprehensive programme plan in the behavioural and social areas.

Some of the new developments in computer-managed instruction (McLeod, 1985) and allied areas, make such a recording system possible and also provide opportunities for staff to know intimately the details of programming that are necessary. Further, the availability of these records to the client or client's representative is extremely important, for without a knowledge of where the individual is going, self-image, motivation and development of skills is unlikely to occur effectively. The type of process that needs to be recorded obviously includes some of the items mentioned in the chapter on assessment. However, following the model put forward a variety of daily measures which relate to fluctuation of performance and output, along with clinical notes concerning primary and secondary positive and negative impacts, plus the reaction to the individual to unfamiliar or new situations, are extremely important.

Rule systems

There is a danger that all new methods which become popular are prone to written procedure and rule domination. The written manual may provide for information and correct procedure, but it can stifle the flexibility to design or amend programmes for individual need. Although frequently urged in North America as a means of counteracting the path to litigation, should accident or improper service occur, there is evidence (Marlett, 1986) that the most successful and flexible managers are those who do not have large and detailed procedure manuals. In order to develop new procedures it may be necessary to pilot them using visual or pictorial processes. Excessive verbal content at this stage may be very limiting even though bureaucracies require detailed and precise verbal systems. The generative stage described in the model is one that often requires or involves lowered verbal systems, which must be tolerated during the piloting of new projects. The precise verbalization comes later. Static and written rule systems inhibit this process.

When rules are brought into systems of rehabilitation their proponents and designers must recognize that their primary purpose is to serve clients. The effectiveness of a new rule system is directly related to its outcome with clients. Many of the rules that are brought into effect by local authorities and others are often rules of protection and care. Sometimes, for example, it is not recognized that individuals need to live in a home-like environment with opportunities for work and training which enable them to function effectively. Such rules may involve, for example, the number of individuals who live in a particular community house, access to various parts of the home, privacy, and the need for training in terms of home living knowledge and experience. Sometimes rules relate to fire risks, hazards, or possible insurance claims which could arise because of negligence. Rule systems that are generated by, and put the onus on, staff control, for reasons of protection, may not always be in the interests of the individuals.

There is a tendency amongst agencies to proliferate rules and put them in writing. Such rules when posted do not make for a convenient home-like atmosphere, especially in residential settings. They provide an over-rigid structure system which does not encourage or allow clients to develop and explore, or form new associations, without feelings of anxiety or fear of punishment. Wherever possible, within the behavioural rehabilitation area, written rules should be kept to a minimum.

On the other hand it should be recognized that staff frequently misunderstand or conveniently forget rule systems. Indeed, new ideas and suggestions may need to be repeated by managers many times before staff accept their existence. In the experience of the authors, innovative systems cause many staff concerns and their application may not be understood. The behaviour is merely following the unfamiliarity effect. Staff may regress to a former system to the extent they may suggest the new arrangements have not come into effect or are non-existent. Alternatively they may be seen as unworkable or not as desirable as procedures in 'the old days'. The new system may confuse staff and clients alike. But behavioural regression is a phenomenon of human beings, not just clients! This suggests that regular meetings and discussions between staff over issues of this type are extremely important. The issue relates to the myth system referred to earlier, and to feelings of team leadership and co-operation in working with specific clients. The new system must be derived from staff thinking and practice. An effective manager ensures that it takes place, and staff co-operate because they personally developed the structure and usually are invested in the desired results. Changing systems or rules is like changing behaviour. Need for change can often be seen or understood, but initiating people into a process of actually changing their behaviour to improve a particular outcome is far more difficult (e.g. 'I know we should do it differently, but we cannot because . . . gets in the way'). An insightful manager may apply this suggested model by proposing the need for staff to consider ways to make changes but not demanding immediate suggestions for improvement or compliance. He or she then returns to the question of initiating change, often to find that staff will have thought about it and devised practical solutions. Compliance then comes more naturally.

When rules are set they must take into account the need for future as well as present performance. The opportunities afforded by any system must always be devised in such a manner that the individual can generalize knowledge to other situations. For example, training of visually impaired individuals to make their way around a kitchen with safety, but with ability to recognize placement of dishes, food, oven, etc., must use the same techniques that are employed in their own home for when they return to that home. This provision is essential. If rules are provided for protection of an individual, and thus prevent experience of a condition which prevails at home, then the rule either prevents effective training or there must be modification in the home. The rule must take into account the aim of a process. In the present example an effective rule system could only be developed when staff have knowledge of the home situation. The issue here is whether agencies are designed to provide training and experience, or a family-like atmosphere with care and protection as the major priority.

Staff and client relations

Change may come about through other mechanisms. For example, change in environment, through movement of staff or clients, may produce major effects in the rehabilitation process. The effect of such changes, regardless of cause, is partly dependent on the applied philosophy of the agency. Of course, staff change their jobs and move on to new environments. Sometimes staff are moved for the convenience of the staff or for the convenience of the management team. Programme philosophy and practical needs of the clients, as perceived by the clients, must be taken into account when moving or appointing staff. The effects of staff movement must be discussed with staff and managers during their training.

Rigid duty rosters which may relate to union contracts, not client need, may also affect client perceptions of the environment, and may interfere with training requirements and client growth. As we learn more about client needs, so union and management rules must adjust to absorb these requirements. This is a *sine qua non* of rehabilitation. For example, the strict adherence to duty hours or specific tasks and routines, by particular staff, may not help to create a supportive home-like atmosphere. Such job contracts may relegate training or experience to specific hours of the day, which may militate against client rehabilitation.

It is recognized that changes can have adverse effects on client behaviour and recovery. When one is dealing with long-term rehabilitation, or short-term but very difficult rehabilitation, it can be expected that clients will make strong emotional bonds with one or more staff members. Very often this 'bonding' is reciprocated, and although little attention is generally paid to this within training systems, it does provide an instance where counselling and support often needs to be provided to client and staff. The process is recognized in psychoanalytic and counselling situations, but not, as a rule, in other one-to-one or small group programmes. 'Bonding' and personal development are very important aspects of rehabilitation, for without them motivation, self-image and the ability to try new systems under stress cannot easily occur. It should be remembered that rehabilitation can provide a daily if not hourly brush with situations which are difficult, even traumatic, for the individual. Familiarity and stress effects have been clearly outlined. Change in staff or staff routines may be seen in client performance as a decrement in behaviour.

The ideal is 'only change one thing at a time'. Certain changes are desirable, or should be tried, but rehabilitation knowledge suggests this should only be done when the reasons and motives have been explained to clients, along with the possible effects. Rearrangements should be detailed to client and relatives, to help ensure the individual continues unimpeded, or with as minimal negative effects as possible.

Staff often believe the client cannot understand or be concerned. Regardless of disability, attempts at explanation should be made, not in writing, but orally and, wherever possible, visually. Videotapes of foreign procedures or work or community environments can be helpful, and in this context assistance in 'bonding' to the situation can be promoted by assisting the individual to imagine himself in the situation. In this way the process is visualized and the individual is assisted in dealing with the personal emotions of the situation. As a final message a written and simple statement may be helpful. Consulting the client gives status and may result in additional and helpful suggestions.

The effects of unfamiliarity upon training and on behaviour have been described, and it is suggested that more simple verbal systems and tactile support systems are likely to be required. Ley and Spelman (1965) have given eloquent examples of patient confusion over oral statements by general medical practitioners. McLeod and Brown (1976) have documented information loss amongst the clients of social workers and counsellors, where verbal information has been provided to developmentally handicapped adults. An implicit understanding of such processes for emergencies, where of course stress is involved, is observed in the airline industry. For the English traveller 'Boucler les Ceintures' causes more delay than a visual image of a lighted seat belt sign, accompanied by the single sound of a bell. Visual and, indeed, tactile stimuli (touching and pointing) can be very effective teaching mechanisms. Yet visual, and particularly tactile, stimuli between staff and client also help to foster a nurturant relationship—one that, in some instances, can lead to major upset, even disaster, if not handled with insight and care. Tactile and visual components are the basic components of emotional relationships. For example, in a recent study (Brown, Bayer and MacFarlane, 1985), an account is given of one young man who was removed from a residential home unit because of affectional relations which developed between him and a staff member. The arbitrary removal of that individual to a new home resulted in elective mutism!

Some general recommendations follow:

1. Staff may need to be attached for long periods of time (over several years) to a particular client(s) but not necessarily in the same unit.
2. If staff do move they may be able to transfer from residential to vocational or leisure time units, so that they still remain in contact with the same clients.
3. Staff need to recognize that they cannot, and will not, get on with every client, and they should discuss such concerns with their team leader. A client-staff change should be made where the situation cannot be easily resolved.
4. Staff may form strong emotional relations with clients and vice-versa. This will happen to some degree where there is a positive and individual training or counselling environment. This is not a negative outcome, and can be employed to precipitate greater progress; but the staff member must be aware of the relationship that is developing. Counselling around such matters is very important.
5. Mutual support systems between staff involved are important.
6. If movement of staff is contemplated this should be discussed with the clientele in advance of the changes made and, if necessary, where there is a particular

and critical development between the staff and client, this should be taken into account when the arrangements are made.

Obviously there are occasions when sudden and rapid changes have to occur, but if they do, straightforward explanations about these should be made to the clients as well as other staff members. Other support members who are familiar to the client involved should be available, for the more handicapped the individual, or the more critical the learning situation, the more vulnerable the client to deterioration. The fact that a client cannot hear or speak cannot be taken as evidence that changes will have no effect or can be ignored. These situations demand more help and understanding, with information put forward in an acceptable form. It is a situation which often arises with elderly, mentally deteriorated and very dependent institutionalized clients.

Team models

It is possible to have a variety of teams within an organization, and these teams may be competitive in terms of idea production and innovation. If this is allowed or even promoted in a controlled and constructive fashion, the process begins to serve the needs of different types of clients. Different models are viable within an agency because they meet different behavioural needs. Such flexibility is possible once the type of team strategies outlined above are developed. Furthermore, there needs to be a match between the personality characteristics of specific staff and clients. For example the level of emotional responsiveness of staff may be a relevant variable.

One of the criticisms of such a system is that staff are amalgamated into teams which do not reflect professional departments; for example, there is no social work department, no occupational therapy department, no psychology department. But where individuals are in or relate to multidisciplinary teams there are several advantages. Treatment may be carried out by one or more of these individuals who ensure that their specific skills and knowledge, where appropriate, are imparted to other individuals in the team (often front-line rehabilitation practitioners) so they may carry out the specific training. This is important because certain clients will relate more easily to specific staff members and, further, it conserves a professonal's time if front-line workers can learn the necessary skills. The individual can also receive a more continuous programme over the day with spaced learning, which is critical for many of those undergoing rehabilitation. Thus training can be regular and frequent.

This system also raises the issue of the need for a generic worker, which is discussed in the subsequent chapter. However, specialist professional training, skills and knowledge are important, and it may well be that, in the larger units, individuals need to be bonded into professional departments as well as work with specific teams. This has been done in a number of instances where a lattice model of delivery has been promulgated (McDonald, 1982). Such systems often cause divided loyalties and a number of allied problems. They require much flexibility by staff, since they owe allegiance both to their professional department and also to their functional unit. However, many hospitals and rehabilitation centres are exploring such systems with some success. Provided the guidelines are clear and the allegiances are recognized, then the possibility of transdisciplinary development becomes a reality.

Within such a system the role of the part-time occupational therapist, physiotherapist or social worker becomes critical. Unfortunately, the fact that such individuals may only come for one or two days per week may mean that they are not blended into the team, or are often seen as working for another authority. This is undesirable because these individuals must be seen as part of the team and working for the individual client, with whom they must be familiar. They must be sufficiently well accepted, by the client and staff, that their skills and knowledge are imparted by demonstration as well as practice to other members of the team. Verbal or written statement is insufficient. Because of the nature of information described earlier, psychologists who only provide a written programme for others to follow will not find that their programme is put into effect, or into effect accurately. They must be around to see it put into effect. They are models, monitors and directors. This will be taken by some as an argument against part-time workers, but it only implies that there should be sufficient time amongst professionals, not just to provide assessments and write reports, but to become involved in hands-on training and demonstration of training strategies.

The training workshop

One problem that frequently arises in vocational training and rehabilitation workshops is that the client who is good at carrying out one particular type of activity remains at that activity, because he or she produces a large number of items. This is exacerbated by the fact that many agency employers do not have sufficient funds to hire new staff, and it is difficult for disabled persons to find employment or re-employment. Always of concern, this is now becoming a critical issue. In some cases the trainee or client, unable to progress in or from the agency, becomes an unpaid worker raising money to fund the employment of staff (Brown, Bayer and MacFarlane, 1985). Thus clients in rehabilitation agencies are often one of the few groups raising their own funds for a training from which they cannot largely benefit, because they continue to work at the same job to maintain the funding. Obviously this is iniquitous and authorities concerned with the running of such centres should ensure that it does not happen. This underlines the concern for a re-evaluation of agency philosophy and goals. Adequate arrangements must be made for the progress of the client through the continua described earlier.

The discussion raises the issue of moving a client from a training agency to a sheltered workshop. The latter type of centre is not unreasonable, provided the individual receives a reasonable payment for carrying out the activity, and has received prior long-term training. Further, with change in behaviour the individual should be able to recommence a training system. The issue of rehabilitation as training or sheltered workshop is an extremely important one in terms of government funding. It is relatively easy to provide funds for minimal support, particularly where the agency is generating much of its own funds. It is particularly easy when the individual cannot act as a self-advocate, and self-image and motivation are poor. Indeed the situation becomes even more problematic where the philosophy, goals and procedures are unclear and confound the programme's clarity. The rehabilitation—sheltered workshop issue arises across the western world, and must stand as a major challenge to governments at local, provincial and national levels.

The issue also raises the definition of long-term training. There can be no clear limit of time for rehabilitation, but the model and evidence provided previously suggests that long-term training is much longer than 2—5 years in many clients. The evidence of recovery after a 5-year period for persons with traumatic brain injury, and the known slow process of rehabilitation for mentally handicapped persons, suggests that longer-term opportunities must be provided for individuals receiving training programmes than is currently the case. Again individual assessment and individual programming are essential, but we must remember that our ability to make accurate long-term prediction is very poor.

Placement and follow-up procedures—a management policy

The importance of follow-up procedures for clients who move from one unit to another, from one residence to another, or to work in the community is critical. Considerable evidence has been provided concerning the type of phenomena that will occur under such situations as placement and follow-up in the community. Management should ensure that adequate staff are provided for the periods where sudden changes occur for the client. Often such periods are fraught with stress, resulting in behavioural regression. Unless precautions are taken the likelihood of client failure is very considerable. Once again the ability to deal with stress and panic demands that there is a positive relationship between the staff member and the client, that a familiar bond has been developed which outweighs the difficulties that will occur when unfamiliarity occurs within a situation. Anticipated change for the client requires increase in staff involvement at such times.

Placement in a new home, return to one's own home or a new job should result in programme planning, preparation and familiarization. It should be a period of particular staff alertness, where negative or positive changes in client behaviour are noted. It is a time where upcoming events should be simulated and rehearsed—not once, but until the client has adapted and believes he/she can cope easily. Visual techniques are again important and the work of Dowrick and Biggs (1983) using videotaping represents an effective approach. The staff member must know when to let go or increase support. It is, as described earlier, a time of oscillation and fluctuation in client behaviour, and a time where adjustment in stimulation is needed. Familiar and positive experiences must be introduced as supports to stabilize behaviour.

Unfortunately these needs are often ignored and a simple and bureaucratic approach taken. It may be administratively easier to provide the occasional visit from a worker from another authority who does not know the individual, but oftentimes this will be useless and a waste of funds. It may add to the stress, as the model suggests. Furthermore, action by an unfamiliar worker tends to be taken only when crisis occurs. A familiar worker who knows the individual will pick up nuances that signal impending breakdown, and bring into effect changes which will prevent difficulties becoming more chronic and severe.

Follow-up systems

Follow-up in rehabilitation for many clients who are disabled is a long-term process. It does not relate just to work or short visits to home environments to discuss how the individual is doing in work. It means an intensive follow-up arrangement which ensures that the individual functions in an integrated fashion in all facets of life. This again argues for a generic worker, but a generic worker who is part of a team. Nutrition, physical fitness, leisure time activities, social skills in the community, vocational expertise, relationship with friends and family members and co-workers, are all critical components of rehabilitation success, and need to be maintained and supported.

It is also apparent that no rehabilitation programme can forecast some of the difficulties that clients will get into. Therefore additional training has to be carried out when such difficulties arise. This may mean involving a specialized consultant but, more often than not, such issues are largely practical ones that can be dealt with at time and place of occurrence. There is a need to be able to move rapidly and effectively if major breakdown occurs. For example, when an individual runs into major problems at work it may be necessary to remove him or her from the work environment so that he can undergo a training process again. If the individual is allowed to break down fully, not only will the person's development be limited and the relationship with the family be disturbed, but the employer is likely to be more negative towards the involvement of the person or handicapped persons in general.

It is essential that employment agencies and other persons are informed about the specific needs of the individual and the likely problems which may arise (Vandergoot and Martin, 1986). Further, employing agencies like to know what type of problems may occur in any individual case. Brown et al. (1985) note that one agency was severely criticized by employers for not providing such information. This is another example of familiarity and stress effects. Advance knowledge can equip a firm or factory to deal with such situations through preparation (Young, Rosati and Vandergoot, 1986).

Conclusion

The chapter has provided indications of how a model within the rehabilitation behavioural and educational framework can influence management and administrative structures. The personalization and individualization of services are important. Familiar environments and access to relevant skill training are necessary. Philosophy and goals must go hand-in-hand with practice. Rehabilitation requires an integrated approach, and at the centre of this process is the individual client with his or her personal needs and choices.

CHAPTER TEN

Advocacy and professional practice

Introduction

A consideration of rehabilitation including environment would not be complete without discussion of the developing processes of advocacy and self-advocacy. Such a development fits well with the processes that are now occurring at a behavioural level in terms of training. Furthermore the development of the advocacy system has profound implications for the education and development of professionals. The client has also become the consumer, for the concepts asociated with illness and treatment recede further as the disabled persons or their advocates take a more active role in planning.

Advocacy and client rights

In recent years consumer advocacy and self-advocacy have become major forces in the rehabilitation field. Many parents and others associated with the field of rehabilitation have become intensely aware that clients are not always provided with opportunities to grow, to make choice, and to receive the maximum opportunities which could be offered by society. Over the past 20 years this has resulted in the development of an advocacy system. The awareness that staff members, whatever their profession, though knowledgeable, are biased observers and participants in the rehabilitation process is beginning to be recognized. Because of this, clients often either require an independent advocate, if their voice cannot be heard, or must learn advocacy skills.

The advocacy movement has had growing pains. Sometimes the advocates are forceful individuals lacking in knowledge but rich in compassion for the person for whom they are advocating. Their recommendations may be imprecise and sometimes their approaches unwelcome. At times their approaches are more aggressive than considerate and understanding. But over time greater care has been taken by various organizations interested in developing advocacy, and advocacy training and workshops are now provided in many places. Even so, many agencies and their personnel look askance at such groups, seeing them as a threat and an interference, and project the view that the professional worker 'always knows best'. For these reasons the advocates are often rejected, finding that they are not permitted access to information, and attempts may be made to prevent them speaking to, or on behalf of, the consumer of the service. They may be unwelcome at client meetings even though the client has invited them there.

However, matched volunteer advocates, who become knowledgeable about needs along with the consumer and who have available to them a support group of independent knowledgeable, caring volunteers from the various professions, can represent a strong voice in identifying concerns and needs appropriately at programme meetings. Their involvement can often lead to a consideration of new approaches and new ideas, for the client often needs much time to think through what he or she needs and to come to realistic goals for the future.

Consumers may need help in expressing their concerns. Professionals may need help in learning how to actively listen to the consumer, as well. Agencies often act psychologically, if not legally, as if they are *in loco parentis*. They therefore try to maintain control and become fearful of any independent action taken by the consumer. Yet, rather than being a threat to an agency, such an advocacy approach should be welcomed.

Allied to the development of advocacy in various parts of the world is a recognition of the need for volunteer or allied support for the individual client. In some countries this may be put in the form of a legally recognized arrangement. For example, in parts of Canada and Australia the development by the legislatures of Dependent Adult or Persons Acts, guardianship can, where needed, be provided for the total care of the individual, or for specific areas of incompetence such as money management or home living aspects of life. This enables the individual to develop further through structured supervision and training. The guardian acts *in loco parentis* and may be a lay person or a public representative rather than a professional. Such legislation, in terms of its application, is far from foolproof for although the spirit of the act is to promote independence, it does in fact remove many basic civil and human rights (Dependent Adults Act, Alberta, 1981). Frequently legal authorities do not examine the niceties of dependence and independence, nor understand the nature of incremental growth within the rehabilitation process. Further, those who apply the law may believe in protection rather than training for growth and development. It is important that professional witnesses, who are knowledgeable in the area of environmental aspects of progress and development of disabled persons, share that knowledge with the representatives of the legal process. They can also act as advisors in courts and, where appropriate in agencies, provide consulting advice which may help the client through the legal process by rehearsing or modelling the legal procedure.

Self-advocacy

More recently the concept of self-advocacy has arisen. Although there may be cases where this is inappropriate because the client is not yet capable of this process, it should be recognized that there need to be opportunities for increasing choice and personal control by clients as rehabilitation progresses. While conceding that individual clients must take a major role in decision-making wherever possible, 'too much too early' can lead to lost opportunities. Frequently our rehabilitation systems think in black-and-white terms, either allowing or not allowing choice. In an effective training or rehabilitation programme the ability to make choices gradually becomes critical. This means professional staff members systematically withdrawing their authority and recognizing when they must change from directive to more laissez-faire styles of client management. Such skill requires considerable training.

In both advocacy and self-advocacy, agencies fear interference or assume that the advocates lack adequate knowledge. Yet it must be recognized that the social interaction between client and friend or advocate, and the gradual awareness by the client of his environment and the restrictions he is facing, form an important basis for information. Client need, choice and perceptions about the rehabilitation system in which they are involved are frequently overlooked. Staff need to be sensitized to these issues through demonstration and discussion. Workshops on these particular issues, and the opportunity to be involved in pilot practice, are important. For example some professionals take the opportunity to become advocates of clients in settings which are not associated with the advocate's own agency. Thus they gain opportunities to see the issues from a different perspective and learn to understand what goes on in the client's 'non-rehabilitation life', in addition to becoming aware of the individual's concerns and needs.

Discussion and decision between client and advocate may result in challenges to the rehabilitation system. Certainly this will be a major threat to management and administration, who may be remote from clients and not open to changes within the agency's procedures. However, if the advocacy system is examined openly it can bring about greater sensitivity and increase the diversity of training skills.

Human rights

The above raises the issue of human rights for consumers in services. For example, the adult who is developmentally disabled, who expresses a wish to live with another person of the opposite sex—not in a marriage partnership, but on a trial basis to facilitate physical and social effectiveness, may also be setting challenges to agency and parental authority. In such an example, parents may become very concerned; whereas even if they were concerned with their non-handicapped child, they would not be permitted to play a decision-making role. For the handicapped adult the situation may be much more difficult, with 'stands' being taken by both professional and family representatives. The role of an advocate, who can help support the voice of the individual in a non-emotionally charged manner, may be critically important. This in turn meets specific needs as well as enhancing self-image and promoting later growth.

The regression model is important in this situation, for both staff and family members who disapprove of the client's wishes may, when confronted with a firm stand by the disabled adult, regress in their own behaviour, giving irrational reasons for opposing the client's wishes. Very often visual images are provided of the 'think what will happen if' variety. The problem has a lot to do with control. The agency and family members are in danger of losing it, while the disabled person is seeking to attain it. Loss of control in the situation by parents may lead to regressive behaviour; the client gaining it, if such control is warranted by the situation, will enhance growth. The assumption is that the client is not in a position to judge. If reasons are advanced through an advocate, even though some risk-taking is involved, such requests should be looked at seriously.

Professional staff should be trained to have insight into their own behaviour. They must be able to change their roles from directive to supportive when the situation demands. They must also have the skills to support, advise and encourage parents or relatives to examine their own, as well as the client's, motivation. This may mean the use of visual and other concrete examples of behavioural interaction. A new situation is unfamiliar and its temporally abstract quality means that it may be rejected for non-valid reasons.

Examples of consumer rights

The following examples illustrate the issue. In one case two women elected to live together; one agreed to carry out a job in the community, while the other did not wish to gain employment but to provide support in the home by cooking, cleaning and shopping. The latter person had major physical deficits and also had problems relating to physical appearance which made it difficult for her to obtain a job. The potential partners related well to each other, but the first individual, although of low cognitive level and poor home living skills, was capable and keen to undertake employment. In this case advocacy was important to enable an agency to recognize that a partnership at this time might be very effective, and that requirements for vocational placement for both persons were probably inappropriate. The agency had some difficulty in recognizing that a non-vocational role would be socially and practically viable. The two individuals have now lived as a partnership for many years in the community, although they both are, in different ways, severely handicapped.

A further example involved a man and a woman who suffered from major physical disabilities and were unable to cope in a home environment without considerable support from professionals. They needed support in washing and dressing, and were restricted in terms of physical movement. By joining in a partnership, where the male could assist the female in washing and dressing and each could help the other in a wide range of domestic skills, a viable partnership could lead to a reasonable degree of independence. In this particular case staff and relatives were worried because of sexual connotations and expected social disapproval, yet the individuals concerned, because of their own strengths, advocated and insisted on their right to make this choice as adults.

Although there are examples of disabled persons who are able to assert their wishes, many more could do so if they were provided with advocacy support. It must be recognized that those who have authority by position, or through the disability of those for whom they are responsible, frequently fear the loss of control. Relationships are balances between attempts at control, and independence. This process is evidenced in normal family relations. Many disabled persons, because they are more dependent and encouraged to be dependent, have difficulty in asserting their needs and wishes, especially when still young adults.

It should be recognized that professionals, although they have skill and knowledge, do not have the right to make choices for the individual when that individual is in a position to advocate and argue extensively for self-choice. Many professionals enter rehabilitation because they are caring people; they wish to nurture and protect. But these characteristics on their own may be a liability unless they can be balanced by skills and pleasure in seeing people grow to independence during which clients divorce themselves from the rehabilitation process. The judgement is a subtle one for, as we have indicated, it is only with growth and development that people have enough information for valid choice. It must also be recognized that each of us has the right to choose even though we may be wrong. One of the rights often denied handicapped persons is the right to make a mistake, and it is through such mistakes that much learning and adjustment can take place. It is the interaction between the advocate, the clients advocating for themselves, and the professional worker that realistic goals and attainment can be developed. However, this means that the professional member must have insight into his or her own attitudes to control, prior to taking on the role of rehabilitation practitioner. Thus self-awareness, and the learning of advanced counselling skills by the practitioner, are critical components in professional training. Role-playing, which is videotaped and examined by a skilled leader, is desirable, and provides staff with opportunities to understand the processes involved in personal choice.

Unfortunately few practitioners ask what are the internal feelings, choices and wishes of disabled individuals. The recent interest in cognitive psychology, and the greater recognition of the role of self-image and self-awareness, are making practitioners more cognizant of the fact that we have not tapped the wide and diverse range of emotional resources of many clients.

Unfortunately some disabled persons, because they may be passive and have poor self-image, are not in a position to assert their choice and rights. For example a young handicapped female, who was doing poorly at vocational work, attended a series of personality and sexuality awareness sessions. During these sessions she showed considerable anxiety and concern. A skilled female counsellor who noted this invited the person to individual sessions and carefully elicited experiences involving sexual abuse, which had been sustained over many years. In this particular case self-image was very poor, and the individual found it difficult to function effectively in any role. The counsellor, by dealing with these issues, enabled the person to assert gradually her own rights, and come to grips with the former abuse, and its attendant negative self-image. This eventually resulted in rapid and dramatic increases in vocational performance. The example illustrates that vocational disability may not be related to vocational ineptitude. However the issue was first raised through counselling procedures involving considerable visual content.

The points raised do not suggest that professionals or parents 'give in' to everything that the disabled person requests. As we have indicated, choice is based on a knowledge continuum. As one reaches new levels of performance, so one questions and chooses at a higher level. One's reach for new information, and attempts to make choices, outreaches one's grasp of situations; but it is only with such an attempt that one can begin to grasp further development.

Positive advocacy enables disabled people to understand themselves more clearly and represent their wishes more cogently. Yet there are many times when agencies, parents and their adult children come into conflict. At a recent agency Annual General Meeting some clients asked to put forward a motion to change the name of the society to one that represented themselves first and their handicap second. They wished it to be a society for people with disabling conditions, rather than a society for a disability. Because of advocacy, which included advice to enable the clients to express their opinions, and through a helpful chairman, who encouraged them to speak up, one particular disabled person became an effective spokesman. The agency meeting had to be recessed shortly afterwards because parents became angry, saying it was the parents' agency, not the children's, because they had formed the society. The debate became so fierce that the Chairman of the Board was accused of being partisan. Fortunately a recess, further background of diplomacy and discussion resulted in a task force being formed with representation from all the parties concerned. Within a few months the society's name was changed. Without the support of an advocate, and a sensitive chairman who would listen to someone who stammered and had difficulty in expressing views, such a change would not have been possible. One might argue the result was only a change in a few words. However, it makes a difference in terms of disabled people being recognized as individuals, with rights to assert, opportunities for self-image to grow, and chances to play a role in the development of the structures which are said to be there to help.

This type of situation is going to confront us increasingly as new agencies are developed in the fields, for example, of ageing and brain injury, and could become prevalent as the new privatized organizations gain momentum. Agencies that have power and money, or agencies which are large, bureaucratic and remote, tend not to have time for individual concerns. Yet these concerns are the essence of rehabilitation education for, as has been indicated earlier, without consulting the clients, and without involving them in the total process as decision-makers, there can be few behavioural or social advances.

Consulting the consumer about programmes

In all of these processes it is important to take into account the needs and wishes of the consumer of the service. It has not been popular to consult the client in detail about personal concerns, wishes and needs. Such consultation is critical, as is consultation with family members. One of the major reasons for the inefficiency of particular rehabilitation programmes is that very little information is taken from clients, who are seen as disabled and are thus not considered able to provide appropriate comment. It must not be assumed that parents necessarily know what is best for their offspring. Judgements are often made in relation to the verbal competency of the client or family, whereas many handicapped persons have considerable non-verbal skills and can conceptualize their concerns if given time and an appropriate medium for experience. This is also true of many non-handicapped children. A study by Brown et al. (1985) shows that clients and their closest family members or sponsors know the areas in which the individual is deficient, and frequently this is correlated with deficiencies in the agency programme.

Data suggest that the areas of leisure time and social competence are valued very highly by clients and family members. Yet frequently these areas are not dealt with other than in a formal manner within the agencies concerned. Even in day or general hospitals concentrating on psychiatric care, scant attention may be given to home and community management within the individual's home environment. In programmes for elderly persons the same concerns arise. In some cases occupational therapy does not relate to meaningful activities, leaving the individual unable to cope with home management deficits, which were part of the original complex of presenting problems. Two related concerns arise from this:

1. The disease model often takes pre-eminent position, i.e. if we cure the disease the symptoms will go away. Thus it is assumed that a cure for depression will enable the individual to cope at home, or medical treatment of brain injury will overcome difficulties the individual has in the community. If the individual does reman physically or mentally disabled, the individual will need to learn at home, but will not generally be provided with a comprehensive learning programme. The rehabilitation education concept recognizes an environmentally induced symptomatology. Thus we underline the environment-management model in rehabilitation.

2. The disease entity model results in labelling. Thus there are the disabled, the handicapped, the elderly, the mentally ill and epileptic, etc. This approach depersonalizes the client—the individual becomes the disease. The familiarity model directs us to personalize the individual. This sometimes makes the rehabilitation situation more difficult for many staff from an emotional perspective. But it is the proper infusion of emotional concern which is critical in an effective rehabilitation model. Individualization and familiarization processes help to promote this. Unless this can occur the individual client is given treatment rather than, from a psychological perspective, the chance to participate in a development process. Generally it is left to the individual to personalize or make the programme his or her own, and therefore use and adapt it to his or her own personal needs. This personalization is recognized by the People First Movement (Park, 1986).

Self-advocacy, the client as programme designer

Clients must be consulted on an equal basis in programmes, for they know much about their own functioning, and it is necessary to make use of their internal motivation and knowledge in planning for behavioural change. There are particular occasions when this is critical—during initial assessment, development of the individual rehabilitation plan, and at various stages of change and follow-up; preferably in advance of the change process. Yet this must be done with a recognition that the individual's level of performance may require a highly structured programme where opportunities to learn systems are critical. Choice comes on a graduated basis, and must be related to the level of functioning of the person involved. Again such decisions should not be made arbitrarily, but through the knowledge base of the team concerned.

In various fields of disability, including, to some extent, amongst mildly mentally handicapped individuals, a self-advocacy movement has grown. Many young adults are unhappy remaining in a home environment or receiving special aid and support within schools. They see themselves as part of an adult community, which requires work and adult living conditions, and many of them wish to live on their own. The self-help movement has arisen to deal with such concerns (see Biklen, 1983). With this development many handicapped persons have recognized that they are people first and only secondly have a disability. They do not see their disability as an illness. Thus there is a growing negative feeling towards a medical model which still looks to hospitalization and clinical and medical treatment as the answer to physical disabilities (see Gliedman and Roth, 1980; Marlett, 1987). That current approaches to disability have not dealt with some of the major concerns is underlined by the fact that amongst physically disabled students of considerable ability (e.g. those who attend universities in Canada), almost none of them have had after-school employment, nor have they had summer jobs compared with their non-disabled peers (Marlett, 1987).

With the development of self-advocacy there have been attempts to start associations of disabled persons for disabled persons. Gradually, in the more advanced areas of rehabilitation, there is a recognition that rehabilitation personnel are partners with each person with a disability rather than controllers and experts.

On the one hand they recognize the importance of ethological aspects of handicap, seeing disability as a process of social intervention and social advocacy. On the other hand, because such movements are fraught with difficulties and ethological approaches are complex, it is not believed the self-advocacy movement, or even the advocacy movement, can be the sole answer to the issue of rehabilitation. Nevertheless, the development of such movements is critical, for they involve an assertion of personal rights. A recent example is in Canada where the new Charter of Rights and Freedoms may give considerable leverage to disabled persons to see themselves as equal and able to challenge disadvantaged conditions.

Mitchell (1986) has provided a wide model of environmental conditions in disability based on Bronfenbrenner's ethological discussion. It is in this context that a model such as that described by Marlett (1987) can be employed for many people with disabilities. It provides a system whereby the individual, through a simplified verbal process, can examine some of the problems which he or she is facing. Marlett argues for the identification of what she refers to as constraints through self-examination. By using simple verbal terms to provide a rather more concrete approach to counselling situations, where the dominant role is taken by the disabled person, a list of constraints are developed such as social barriers, experiential and physical limitations, situational and personal constraints. A detailed analysis is made of the environment as well as the individual's personal interaction with that environment. The individuals with counselling support select areas on which they wish to work and can construct, through service brokerage or other means, services, guidance and a methodology to deal with these issues. It is important to recognize that such an approach is a significant one, and bound to have a place in future services. It provides a practical counselling approach which sees the issues not as classical handicap, but as problem-solving situations which can be mediated by the disabled person.

This approach fits well with the model that has been advocated, but on its own may have many limitations, and it is important that advocacy approaches identify the strengths and weaknesses of such a formulation. It is extremely important that the self-advocate, or the advocate, recognizes and identifies the needs for structured support and intervention. In the model put forward, those who are least able to identify their needs and limitations will be those who reject the involvement of planned professional approaches. For example, those who come from the more adverse social backgrounds, or have suffered the greatest abuse, are likely to be those less ready to employ the open-ended model described by Marlett.

If, however, the model is to be effective, there will be times when structure will need to be imposed. It is not always possible to leave individuals to their own resources. Frustration, failure, or an incomplete grasp of the system may lead to various kinds of breakdown. The open situation where the advocate or self-advocate makes all the decisions, or is left with advice alone, will not work in a number of instances. The model proposed indicates there is professional as well as supporting oscillation with people progressing and regressing. There is therefore during regression a greater need for structure to be provided. Yet we also argue that professionals must also support the advocacy model with a recognition that we are not dealing just with disease entities or disabilities, but with growth and change within the social community. In order to do this effectively practitioners will have to be retrained and programmes redesigned.

There are already instances of self-advocacy programmes in effect, yet at the present time there is little in the way of funding to evaluate them. Ideally, such programmes should be evaluated on a conjoint basis, as suggested by Westwood (1986). The evaluation is carried out through a process of design development and agreement between the proposing agency and the funders. In the present case, however, we recommend that one other equal party being involved is the disabled person or his or her advocate. This must not be taken to mean that only a few or a minority of disabled people will be represented, but a very wide range of persons, in terms of the descriptors used in this book. They will include most of those with mental illness, a large number of those suffering from disability resulting from ageing, a wide range of mentally handicapped persons, and of course a wide range of those suffering from problems of delinquency.

It must be recognized that as the extended family patterns begin to shift within western culture, and the supports that were available when families were less mobile, a professional group of counsellors, psychologists, social workers and mental health workers are taking their place. An alternative to these professionalized supports has been the massive growth of self-help support groups. It is estimated that there are thousands of groups organized in North America (Biklen, 1983). Such groups reject professional models of caring and are becoming the personalized support substitutes, not only for many groups of people with different disabilities, but also for people going through various life transitions (e.g. single parenting, widowers).

Outreach programmes

The above discussion leads to the importance of outreach programmes. Much of what has been suggested in the rehabilitation model requires that training take place in realistic, familiar and natural environments. Most of our rehabilitation agencies are set within four walls, often in hospital environments or in similar agencies where they are seen as consistent with schools or other places of learning. However, in recent years there has been a move to help adults with a mental handicap, for example, to attend community colleges. This represents an adult learning environment and it is within the normal community (Hutchinson, 1983). If the programmes that are provided are given by staff who know little about disability, or by individuals who try to replicate a model which is a watered-down version of technical or academic education, then such ventures are likely to fail (Brown, 1984b). It seems to us essential, when such models are used, that the body of knowledge in rehabilitation education, using the continuum described earlier, be incorporated. Moreover, and probably most importantly, much of the training should be integrated in the individual's local community and home environment.

It seems likely that parents, sponsors and others will not have the time, the ability, and sometimes the inclination to carry out rehabilitation training in their own environments for a long period of time (Brown and Hughson, 1980). Indeed an examination of rehabilitation inadequacies listed by parents in the Brown *et al.* (1985) study showed that the skills required were frequently not taught in the home by parents, although there were no physical or financial reasons why this should not have been done (e.g. changing light bulbs, budgeting one's money, buying or taking part in the buying of one's clothes). Families are frequently supportive, often providing opportunity and encouraging skill practice by the individual, as long as guidance, support and initial learning procedures are provided by the rehabilitation system. However, they may not, because of the long-term stress and emotional involvement, become major teachers.

Outreach worker and management systems

Proper guidance, support and teaching cannot generally be given effectively in an agency far away from home (Brown, Hughson and Nemeth, 1981). It requires the involvement, within the home and the local community, of an outreach worker who can work with the client in the individual's home environment, thus demonstrating what can be done. Such a system requires a broad knowledge base and understanding of the individual situation, as well as an awareness and sensitivity to family structure (Mitchell, 1986). In our experience such a model is very important within the areas of mental illness, geriatrics, mental retardation, learning disabilities, visual impairment and other disabling conditions.

This approach requires the development of a new form of outreach worker, and involves a wide range of training which has not been envisaged at this time. Furthermore, it breaks entirely with the type of hierarchical process which has been employed in the past, for such professional persons must be in charge of their own work, and be able to carry out training programmes in the way they consider fit. This assumes a high level of professional training. They may need to obtain the assistance of a consultant, but in this model the consultant is an advisor and demonstrator, not a director of the programme. The person who organizes the programme is the outreach worker. The person who eventually directs the programme is the client. Such a system can be effectively brought about by current changes which are under way. For example, effective privatization of rehabilitation could lead to a brokerage model where the client or the sponsor could contract for specific services. However, without an effective philosophy for rehabilitation and well-trained staff, such a privatization process may only lead to new forms of institutionalization.

The type of hierarchical models which worked well in the past were those where senior staff supervised the behaviour and activity of more junior staff. In the situation described above this is impossible, and therefore the level of training that needs to be carried out prior to professional practice is critical. When using such a model the reporting system is different. It must relate to the individual rehabilitation plan, which must take into account direct feedback from client and sponsor. For they become not only the receivers of service, but the originators of need for service and the service evaluators. This combination is critical to the development of effective service delivery.

Such a system means that staff must be up to date in their knowledge; a knowledge base which is changing on a regular basis. Without this update of knowledge, the gap between research and practice, which has been noted by Mittler (1981b) and others (Clarke, 1977), increases. One of the major ways of overcoming this concern is to ensure that practical in-service units are developed through management structure, that time is allowed for training of staff through visual and direct experience, and advisors and teachers are appointed who can demonstrate to staff the particular methods of instruction at a 'hands-on' level, not just simply by giving verbal direction. Individuals should be given the opportunity of release for further study in universities and colleges, and full use should be made of videotape and computer applications systems for the gaining of knowledge within these particular areas.

The transdisciplinary worker in the client's society

The emergence of transdisciplinary rehabilitation workers is envisaged. These would be individuals who can be employed in a variety of settings with a multidisciplinary range of colleagues, and are capable of working in the community or within specialized rehabilitation agencies. Although arguments have been put forward for a generic worker, and it is believed that the principles of rehabilitation are similar regardless of age and condition, this is not meant to imply that all types of handicapping conditions should be provided with services in the same agency. In fact the thrust is towards the development of the generic community-based worker who is able to provide a wide range of services within community settings. Thus the service is largely individualized.

Such an approach is almost obligatory in major rural areas, such as Canada and Australia, for it is not possible to centralize services unless individuals are removed from their home base and placed in city institutions or agencies. Data in the adult rehabilitation field suggest that individuals often fail when lifestyle is abruptly changed, particularly if after agency training they return to their home environments (Brown, Hughson and Nemeth, 1981). The importance of home support in younger disabled children has also been described by Byrne and Cunningham (1985). But perhaps more important is the wide range of service, community and allied levels of stimuli which impact on the individual and his immediate family (Mitchell, 1986). Loss of these social support and family networks, which often happens to individuals who are institutionalized or sent to agencies for day or residential training, may make it impossible for the individual to later take his or her place in the normal adult community. The reasons for this have been discussed in previous chapters.

The development of programme workers must be linked to a comprehensive system which has as its highest priority individualized training, strategies and programmes which are supported by an effective model, for disabled individuals (a) take a long while to rehabilitate, (b) frequently suffer high levels of stress during the recuperative process, and (c) deteriorate due to ageing or other factors; but often they can function in the community with a reasonable level of quality of life with the support and occasional intervention of such workers. Although change (rehabilitation) takes a long time, intensive periods of training may be for short, specific periods. The development of such services is critical. It is critical because the existing approaches are not working effectively, and because the numbers of individuals with physical and geriatric conditions who require support and nurture are increasing.

Existing personnel

In order to make the proposed system work effectively it is apparent that existing professionals will need retraining at philosophical as well as practical levels. Their energies must be redirected. The importance of a sense of mission and the impact of a positive belief system on services has been ably described by Neufeldt (1986), and the impact of negative views about rehabilitation is extremely damaging.

The management structures involved have been discussed in the previous chapter, but the changes required relate to the need to ensure that within society it is possible for personnel to collaborate with families and the client in the family milieu. This frequently means that group counselling and demonstration are required, because it is essential to change the attitudes of family members, not just direct rehabilitation to the obviously affected client. As indicated earlier, such changes result not just from verbal counselling, but from direct demonstration of what can be done in terms of training within the home environment. Very often such demonstrations are simple, make use of baseline assessment and then take a key task, of a social or behavioural nature, that is perceived as contributing to quality of lifestyle environment and will support the individual within his or her home. This might mean learning a simple task like washing one's hair. It may be learning how to dress, or it may mean carrying out grocery shopping within the community. The first demonstration needs to be simple, related to baseline attainments, and easily learned and performed, but it must have value in the individual's and the family's eyes.

The model is one of individualized service, based on a framework that recognizes variability amongst clients within a rehabilitation system (Gunzburg, 1968; Brown, 1984a). Such variability can only be met if there are individual programme plans (IPP) and personnel who interface their programme skills with opportunities within the community. This implies that the management and administrative structures in government and in local services must be flexible in order to adapt to the needs of such a programme. The need is not for large amounts of capital funds, but rather for operational funds to be provided on a long-term basis. It is essential, in countries where large amounts of voluntary fund-raising is carried out, to recognize that this fund-raising must be directed towards such purposes. This is much more abstract a concept than providing buildings and buses with people's name-plates emblazoned upon them!

There must be outreach evaluation of such services, and that evaluation must, to a large degree, involve the client and sponsor (Shaw, 1984). This alone can ensure some programme consistency. The availability of independent others to assess the value of programmes, by taking into account the requirements of the individuals concerned, is also important. However a collaborative model of evaluation between sponsor (often government) and direct service (often private agency) and the consumer (client) is a form of evaluation that can benefit all sides, and result in effective changes in service delivery which all parties agree upon (Westwood, 1986). One advantage in this tripartite evaluation is that it involves one major shift. It removes the secrecy of evaluation results and makes them available to present and potential consumers of the service.

It must also be recognized that individuals have continuing needs. The availability of generic support systems for individuals who continue to run into problems is essential, particularly in relation to practical issues. This means that individualized programmes of a practical and supportive nature over a lifetime are frequently required. This is a concept not accepted within our social system, but the increasing complexity of life makes such a service mandatory and recognizes the vulnerability of need by all citizens.

Although this book has not gone into the cost-effectiveness of such procedures it is suggested that, in terms of quality of life and need within a community, the provision of services within home environment, rather than on a mass basis within institutions or agencies, is to be highly applauded. Support systems will be required in local areas, and already services are beginning to develop in this regard; yet, as indicated earlier, consumers have little say in terms of need, but these needs are beginning to be very clearly expressed and well-articulated from clients. This again underlines the recognition of intrapersonal processes and their importance in directing rehabilitation (Brown, Bayer and MacFarlane, 1985).

There are new ventures under way which are beginning to change the nature of rehabilitation education. Technical aids and the involvement of computers in the field of management and education create more options for many people. These innovations provide the opportunity for many to function from a home base. Professionals and consumers, through data communication systems, can live or be located within a specific area and, in so doing, change the focus in the local community by helping to mediate and model change both in society and in the life of people with disablities.

The rehabilitation model provides possibilities for interleaving information systems so that there are comprehensive data on each client both over time and as he or she moves across geographical areas. Clients, wherever possible, should have access to such data systems, and should have the ability to insert their requirements, needs, hopes and fears into such a system so these can be taken into account. The development of multi data and information systems is now occurring (e.g. Walter Dinsdale Disability Information Service Centre, Calgary, Canada). Such systems will not only be accessible to consumers, but operated by consumers.

One danger of such a system is that individual workers may become isolated in their activities. In-service training, release time, programme and professional meetings all help to overcome the disadvantages. Further, the professional society which provides information on resources and rehabilitation approaches is now developing complex data networks which can be accessed from a home environment (Marlett, 1986). Many professional associations make continuing education a requirement for continued membership of the professional society. This should occur for rehabilitation personnel, and is now becoming more possible through consolidation of information.

It is obvious, in developing such a system, that much of the model needs to be worked out in practice. It is apparent that it does offer opportunities for the individual to deal with a wide range of issues concerned with self-image, motivation and individualized knowledge base. The possibility of such a programme serving the client is considerable, but this will only work if adequate relief services are available. For example, individual clients may need to leave home for brief periods to ensure that adequate training takes place. Thus the need for a local and specialized environment where training can be carried out over several weeks or months will still be required to provide training in very specific types of skills (e.g. mobility training for the visually impaired person). But to be effective it should be located with the home area of the individual, a process which is being developed by the Canadian National Institute for the Blind (Brown, 1985).

Concluding comments

This chapter has attempted to look at some important changes that are taking place in terms of the perception of rehabilitation as a behavioural and educational process in which the disabled person plays a highly personal role. His or her needs as expressed by the individual or through an advocate must come to play an important part in service delivery. This is not to devalue the role of the professional, but to indicate that it must move from technical competence to sophisticated recognition of the changing nature of behaviour in the rehabilitation process, and a realization that the practitioner role changes dramatically at times, in terms of the amount of structure and programme direction that is required.

It is also recognized that a truly sophisticated service must utilize the community environment to a much greater degree, thus moving the professional from an agency-based mode of operation to the individual home, local community and workplace.

The effects of this change, if viewed at a comprehensive and transdisciplinary level, will alter the nature of training of rehabilitation practitioners, and raise it to a much more professional level, involving a philosophy from which technical programme needs can be organized into an effective delivery service. Some indications of change in professional education are indicated. In our view the development of the rehabilitation educator at a professional level is now beginning to emerge as some university programmes develop a range of transdisciplinary education.

However, none of this will be effective unless the rehabilitation practitioner recognizes the central and active role of the individual who has the disability. A blend of organized intervention has to take place which capitalizes on the development of positive self-image, environmental resources and the application of sophisticated and generic rehabilitation services which employ behavioural, social, educational and health resources.

References

Abramson, L.Y., Seligman, M.E., and Teasdale, J.D. (1978). Learned helplessness in humans: critique and reformulation, *Journal of Abnormal Psychology*, **87**, 49–74.

Achenbach, T.M., and Edelbrock, C.S. (1982). *Manual for the Child Behavior Checklist and Revised Child Behavior Profile*, Child Psychiatry, University of Vermont, Burlington.

Anastasi, A. (1968). *Psychological Testing*, 3rd edn, Macmillan, New York.

Baine, D. (1978). Criterion references testing and instruction. In J.P. Das and D. Baine (eds), *Mental Retardation for Special Educators*, Charles C. Thomas, Springfield, Illinois.

Barlett, D., and Shapiro, M.B. (1956). Investigation and treatment of a reading disability in a dull child with severe psychiatric disturbances, *British Journal of Educational Psychology*, **26**, 180–90.

Bastian, A.C. (1898), *A Treatise on Aphasia and Other Speech Defects*, Appleton, New York.

Beck, V., Possberg, E., and Brown, R.I. (1977). Recreation leisure time as an integral part of the rehabilitation programming for the mentally handicapped adult, *Research Exchange and Practice in Mental Retardation*, **3**(3), 153–68.

Beck-Ford, V., and Brown, R.I. (In collaboration with Gillberry, M., and Rolf, C.) (1984). *Leisure Training and Rehabilitation: A Program Manual*, Charles C. Thomas, Springfield, Illinois.

Behrmann, M. (1984). *Handbook of Micro Computers in Special Education*, College Hill Press, San Diego, California.

Belsen, W. (1975). *Juvenile Theft: Causal Factors*, Harper & Row, London.

Berg, J. (ed.) (1982). *Perspectives and Progress in Mental Retardation*, Vol. II: *Biomedical Aspects*. Proceedings of the Sixth Congress of the International Association for the Scientific Study of Mental Deficiency, University Park Press, Baltimore, Maryland.

Bernstein, B. (1967). Social structure, language and learning. In A.H. Passow, M. Goldberg and A.J. Taunenbaum (eds), *Education of the Disadvantaged*, Holt, Rinehart & Winston, New York.

Bernstein, G.S., Ziarnik, J.P., Rudrud, E.H., and Czajkowski, L.A. (1981). *Behavioral Habilitation Through Proactive Programming*, P.H. Brooks, Baltimore, Maryland.

Bierer, J., and Evans, R.I. (1969). *Innovations in Social Psychiatry*, Avenue Publishing, London.

Biklen, D.P. (1983). *Community Organizing: Theory and Practice*, Prentice Hall, Englewood Cliffs, New Jersey.

Binet, A., and Simon, T. (1916), *The Development of Intelligence in Children* (translation E.S. Kite), Williams & Wilkins, Baltimore, Maryland.

Blunden, R. (1987). Quality of life in elderly disabled persons. In R.I. Brown (ed.), *Quality of Life and Rehabilitation*, A Series in Rehabilitation Education, Vol. 3, Croom Helm, London (in preparation).

Blunden, R., and Evans, G. (1984). A collaborative approach to evaluation, *Journal of Practical Approaches to Developmental Handicap*, **8**(1), 14–18.

Borgen, W.A., Amundson, N.E., and Biela, P.M. (1987). The experience of unemployment of the physically disabled, *National Consultation on Vocational Counselling* (in press).

Bower, G.H., and Hilgard, E.R. (eds) (1981) *Theories of Learning*, 5th edn, Prentice Hall Inc., Englewood Cliffs, New Jersey.

Brendon, D. (1984). Life at the end of the tunnel?, *Social Work Today*, **16**(5), October.

Bricker, D., Seibert, J.M., and Casuso, V. (1980). Early intervention. In J. Hogg and P.J. Mittler (eds), *Advances in Mental Handicap Research*, John Wiley & Sons, New York.

Bromwich, R. (1981). *Working with Parents and Infants: An Interactional Approach*, University Park Press, Baltimore, Maryland.

Bronfenbrenner, U. (1975). Is early intervention effective? In B. Friedlander, G. Sterritt, and G. Kirk (eds), *Exceptional Infant*, Vol. 3, Brunner/Mazel, New York.

Bronfenbrenner, U. (1976). Is early experience effective? Facts and principles of early intervention: a summary. In A.M. Clarke and A.D.B. Clarke (eds), *Early Experience: Myth and Evidence*, Free Press, New York.

Bronfenbrenner, U. (1979). *The Ecology of Human Development*, Harvard University Press, Cambridge, Massachusetts.

Brown, L., Shiraga, B., Ford, A., Nesbit, J., Van Deventir, P., Sweet, M., York, J., and Loomis, R. (1986). Teaching severely handicapped students to perform meaningful work in nonsheltered vocational environments. In R. Morris and B. Blatt (eds), *Perspectives in Special Education: States of the Art*, Scott, Foresman, Glenview, Illinois.

Brown, R.I. (1964). The effect of visual distraction on perception in subjects of subnormal intelligence, *British Journal of Social and Clinical Psychology*, **1**, 20−8.

Brown, R.I. (1965). The effects of varied environmental stimulation on the performance of subnormal children, *Journal of Child Psychology and Psychiatry*, **7**, 251−61.

Brown, R.I. (1972), Cognitive changes in adolescent slow learners, *Journal of Child Psychology and Psychiatry*, **13**, 183−93.

Brown, R.I. (1981a), Habilitation of handicapped children: some principles which determine practice, *Canadian Association for Young Children Journal*, **7**(2), 29−33.

Brown, R.I. (1981b). Future considerations. In P. Kincaide and R.I. Brown (eds), *Manpower Planning for Serving the Handicapped in the 80's*, Alberta Advanced Education and Manpower, Edmonton.

Brown, R.I. (1984a). Programs and problems in the field of adult rehabilitation. In C.K. Leong and D. Duane (eds), *Understanding Learning Disabilities*, Plenum, New York.

Brown, R.I. (ed.) (1984b). *Integrated Programmes for Developmentally Handicapped Adolescents and Adults*, A Series in Rehabilitation Education, Vol. 1, Croom Helm, London.

Brown, R.I. (ed.) (1985). *Evaluation of the Adjustment to Blindness Program*, Report to the Canadian National Institute for the Blind, Alberta Region.

Brown, R.I. (ed.) (1986a). *Management and Administration of Rehabilitation Programmes*, A Series in Rehabilitation Education, Vol. 2, Croom Helm, London (College Hill Press, San Diego, California).

Brown, R.I. (1986b), A study of leisure activities in Arab children (in preparation).

Brown, R.I. (1986c), Overt responses and reading difficulties—delays in reading time (in preparation).

Brown, R.I., and Hughson, E.A. (1980). Training of the Developmentally Handicapped Adult, Charles C. Thomas, Springfield, Illinois.

Brown, R.I., and Semple, L. (1970). Effects of unfamiliarity on the overt verbalization and perceptual motor behaviour of nursery school children, *British Journal of Educational Psychology*, **40**(3), 291−8.

Brown, R.I., Bayer, M.B. and MacFarlane, C. (1985). *Rehabilitation Programs Study*, Report to Health and Welfare, Canada (Grant No. 4558-29-4).

Brown, R.I., Bayer, M.B., and MacFarlane, C. (1987). Preliminary results from the Rehabilitation Programs Study, *National Consultation on Vocational Counselling*, (in press).

Brown, R.I., Hughson, E.A., and Nemeth, S. (1981). *The Total Life Program: A Study into* the Feasibility of Community Based Services for Developmentally Handicapped Persons in a Rural Area, Report to Health and Welfare, Canada.

Bryant, P., and Bradley, L. (1985). Children's Reading Problems, Blackwell, Oxford.

Byrne, E.A., and Cunningham, C.C. (1985). The effects of mentally handicapped children on families—a conceptual review, Journal of Child Psychology and Psychiatry, 26(6), 847–64.

Byrne, E.A., and Cunningham, C.C. (1987). Lifestyle and satisfaction in families of children with Down's syndrome. In R.I. Brown (ed.), Quality of Life and Rehabilitation, Croom Helm, London (in preparation).

Cantrell, M.L., and Cantrell, R. (1980), Ecological problem-solving: a decision making heuristic for prevention–intervention educational strategies. In J. Hogg and P.J. Mittler (eds), Advances in Mental Handicap Research, Vol. 1, John Wiley & Sons, New York.

Clarke, A.D.B. (1977). From research to practice. Presidential Address. In P. Mittler (ed.) Research to Practice in Mental Retardation, Proceedings of the Fourth Congress of the International Association for the Scientific Study of Mental Deficiency, University Park Press, Baltimore, Maryland.

Clarke, A.D.B., and Blakemore, C.B. (1961). Age and perceptual-motor transfer in imbeciles, British Journal of Psychology, 52, 125–131.

Clarke, A.D.B., and Clarke, A.M. (1954). Cognitive changes in the feeble-minded, British Journal of Psychology, 45, 173–9.

Clarke, A.D.B., and Clarke, A.M. (1959). Recovery from the effects of deprivation, Acta Psychologica, 16, 137–44.

Clarke, A.D.B., and Clarke, A.M. (1960). Some recent advances in the study of early deprivation, Journal of Child Psychology and Psychiatry, 1, 26–36.

Clarke, A.D.B., and Clarke, A.M. (1977). Recent Advances in the Study of Subnormality, Mind, London.

Clarke, A.M., and Clarke, A.D.B. (1974). Mental Deficiency: The Changing Outlook, Methuen, London.

Clarke, A.M., and Clarke, A.D.B. (eds) (1976), Early Experience: Myth and Evidence, Open Books, London (Free Press, New York).

Clarke, A.D.B., and Cookson, M. (1962). Perceptual-motor transfer in imbeciles: a second series of experiments, British Journal of Psychology, 53, 321–30.

Clarke, A.D.B., and Hermelin, B.F. (1955), Adult imbeciles: their abilities and trainability, Lancet, 2, 337–9.

Clarke, A.D.B., Clarke, A.M., and Brown, R.I. (1956). Regression to the mean—a confused concept, British Journal of Psychology, 51(2), 105–17.

Cobb, H.V. (1966). The Predictive Assessment of the Adult Retarded for Social and Vocational Adjustment: a Review of the Literature, University of South Dakota, Vermillion, South Dakota.

Cobb, H.V. (1972). The Forecast of Fulfillment, Teachers College Press, New York.

Cohen, J.S., and Dickerson, M.U. (eds) (1983). Hey, We're Getting Old, A Monograph on Aging and Mental Retardation, National Institute on Mental Retardation, Downsview, Ontario.

Coleman, W.L. (1986). Personality and social factors in criminal offenders. Unpublished doctoral thesis, University of Calgary, Calgary, Alberta.

Costello, C.G. (1976). Anxiety and Depression. The Adaptive Emotions, McGill, Queen's University Press, Montreal.

Cunningham, C.C., and Sloper, T. (1977). Parents of Down's Syndrome babies: Their early needs, Child Care Health and Development, 3, 325–347.

Curtis, H. (1975). Biology, 2nd edn, Worth, New York.

Cuvo, A.J. (1979). Multiple baseline design and instruction research: pitfalls of measurement and procedural advantages, American Journal of Mental Deficiency, 84, 219–28.

Das, J.P. (1985). Remedial training for the amelioration of cognitive deficit children. In

A.F. Ashman and R.S. Laura (eds), *The Education and Training of the Mentally Retarded*, Croom Helm, London.

Dellario, P.J., Goldfield, E.A., Farkas, M., and Cohen, M. (1984). Functional assessment of psychiatrically disabled adults. In A.S. Halpern and M.J. Fuhrer (eds), *Functional Assessment in Rehabilitation*, P.H. Brookes, Baltimore, Maryland.

Denham, M.J. (1983). Assessment of quality of life. In M.J. Denham (ed.), *Care of the Long-Stay Elderly Patient*, Croom Helm, London.

Dependent Adults Act (amended 1981) Government of the Province of Alberta, Queen's Printer, Edmonton.

Dobbing, J. (1975). Prenatal nutrition and neurological development. In N.A. Buchwald and M.A.B. Brazier (eds), *Brain Mechanisms in Mental Retardation*, Academic Press, New York.

Douglas, J.W., and Blomfield, J.M. (1949). *Children Under Fire*, Allen & Unwin, London.

Dowrick, P.W. (1978). Suggestions for the use of edited video replay in training behavioural skills, *Journal of Practical Approaches to Developmental Handicap*, **2**,(2), 21−4.

Dowrick, P.W., and Biggs, S.J. (1983). *Using Video, Psychological and Social Applications*, Wiley, Chichester.

Earl, C.J.C. (1961). *Subnormal Personalities: Their Clinical Investigation and Assessment*, Baillière, Tindall & Cox, London.

Edgerton, R. (1967). *The Cloak of Competence*, University of California Press, Berkeley, Los Angeles, California.

Edwards, J., and Giles, H. (1984). Application of social psychology of language: sociolinguistics and education. In P. Tredgill (ed.), *Applied Sociolinguistics*, Academic Press, London.

English, F.W., and Kaufman, R.A. (1975). *Needs Assessment: Focus for Curriculum Development*, Association for Supervision and Curriculum Development, Washington, DC.

Esgrow, C. (1978), Placement and follow-up as part of the rehabilitation process, *Journal of Practical Approaches to Developmental Handicap*, **2**(1), 5−8.

Evans, G., Porterfield, J., and Blunden, R. (1986). Service perspectives from a research perspective: a practical approach. In R.I. Brown (ed.), *Management and Administration of Rehabilitation Programmes*, A Series in Rehabilitation Education; Vol. 2, Croom Helm, London (College Hill Press, San Diego, California).

Ferguson, R., and Larsen, C. (1987). Child life: child care in hospitals. In C. Denholm, R. Ferguson, and A. Pence (eds), *The Practice of Professional Child Care: The Canadian Perspective*, University of British Columbia Press, Vancouver, British Columbia.

Feuerstein, R. (1968). The learning potential assessment device. In B.W. Richards (ed.), *Proceedings of the First Congress of the International Association for the Scientific Study of Mental Deficiency*, pp. 562−5.

Feuerstein, R. (1979). *The Dynamic Assessment of Retarded Performers*, University Park Press, Baltimore, Maryland.

Fewster, G., and Garfat, T. (1987). Residential child care and treatment. In C. Denholm, R. Ferguson, and A. Pence (eds), *The Practice of Professional Child Care: The Canadian Perspective*, University of British Columbia Press, Vancouver, British Columbia.

Finger, S., and Stein, D.G. (1982). *Brain Damage and Recovery*, Academic Press, New York.

Fisher, M.A., and Zeaman, D. (1970). Growth and decline of retardate intelligence. In N.R. Ellis (ed.), *International Review of Research in Mental Retardation*, Academic Press, New York.

Flavell, J. (1963). *The Developmental Psychology of Jean Piaget*, Van Nostrand, Princeton, New Jersey.

Flynn, R.J., Dubac, B. and Vincent, D.R. (1987). Employability assessment of disabled or disadvantaged persons: predictive validity and expectancy tables for two new decision-making aids, *National Consultation on Vocational Counselling* (in press).

Fry, P.S. (1986). *Depression, Stress and Adaptations in the Elderly: Psychological Assessment and Intervention*, Aspen, Rockville, Maryland.

Gaito, J. (1966). *Molecular Psychobiology: a Chemical Approach to Learning and Other*

Behavior, Charles C. Thomas, Springfield, Illinois.

Gibson, D. (1978), *Down's Syndrome: the Psychology of Mongolism*, Cambridge University Press, Cambridge.

Gilligan, C. (1982). *In a Different Voice*, Harvard University Press, Cambridge, Massachusetts.

Gliedman, J., and Roth, W. (1980). *The Unexpected Minority*, Harcourt Brace Jovanovich, New York.

Gold, M.W. (1973). Research on the vocational habilititation of the retarded: the present, the future. In N.R. Ellis (ed.), *International Review of Research in Mental Retardation*, Academic Press, New York.

Golden, C.J. (1981). *Diagnosis and Rehabilitation in Clinical Neuropsychology*, 2nd edn, C.C. Thomas, Springfield, Illinois.

Goldman, P.S. (1975), Age sex and experience as related to the neural basis of cognitive development. In N.A. Buchwald and M.A.B. Brazier (eds), *Brain Mechanisms in Mental Retardation*, Academic Press, New York.

Goldstein, G., and Ruthven, L. (1983). *Rehabilitation of the Brain-Damaged Adult*, Plenum Press, New York.

Grant, W.B. (1971). Some management problems of providing work for the mentally disordered with particular reference to mental handicap. Unpublished M.Sc. thesis, University of Manchester.

Greenough, W.T. (1978). Development and memory: the synaptic connection. In T. Teyler (ed.), *Brain and Learning*, Greylock Publishers, Stamford, Connecticut.

Grunewald, K. (1969). *The Mentally Retarded in Sweden*, National Board of Health and Welfare, Stockholm.

Guastaserro, J.R., and Willer, B.S. (1982). *Community Living Assessment Scale*, Transitional Services Inc., Buffalo, New York.

Gunzburg, H.C. (1960). *Social Rehabilitation of the Subnormal*, Baillière, Tindall & Cox, London.

Gunzburg, H.C. (1968). *Social Competence and Mental Handicap*, Baillière, Tindall & Cassell, London.

Gunzburg, H.C. (1969), *Progress Assessment Chart Manual*, NSMHC, London, and Aux Chandelles, Bristol, Indiana.

Hagin, C. (1982). Language-cognitive disorganization following closed head injury: a conceptualization. In L.E. Trexler (ed.), *Cognitive Rehabilitation: Conceptualization and Intervention*, Plenum Press, London.

Hallahan, D.P., and Kauffman, Y.M. (1978). *Exceptional Children*, Prentice-Hall, Englewood Cliffs, New Jersey.

Halpern, A.D. (1973). General unemployment and vocational opportunities of EMR individuals, *American Journal of Mental Deficiency*, **75**, 123–7.

Halpern, A.S., and Fuhrer, M.J. (1984). *Functional Assessment in Rehabilitation*, P.H. Brooks, Baltimore, Maryland.

Halpern, A.S., Lehmann, J.P., Irvin, L.K., and Heiry, T.J. (1981). *Contemporary Assessment of Adaptive Behavior for Mentally Retarded Adolescents and Adults*, Rehabilitation Research and Training Center in Mental Retardation, University of Oregon, Eugene, Oregon.

Hansen, J.C. (ed.) (1983). *Diagnosis and Assessment in Family Therapy*, Aspen, Rockville, Maryland.

Harlow, H.F. (1961). The development of affectional patterns in infant monkeys. In B.M. Foss (ed.), *Determinants of Infant Behaviour*, Methuen, London.

Hawkridge, D., Vincent, T., and Hales, G. (1985). *New Information Technology and the Education of Disabled Children and Adults*, Croom Helm, London.

Haywood, H.C. (1984). Dynamic assessment: the learning potential assessment device (LPAD). In R.L. Jones (ed.), *Non-discriminatory (High Validity) Assessments: A Casebook*, U.S. Department of Education, Washington, DC.

Haywood, H.C. (1985), Behavior Management and Cognitive Perspective. Lecture to the Calgary Association for Students with Learning Disabilities, Calgary, Alberta.

Hebb, D.O. (1949). *The Organization of Behaviour*, Chapman-Hall, London.

Heber, R., and Garber, H. (1971). An experiment in prevention of cultural-familial mental retardation. In D.A.A. Primrose (ed.), *Proceedings of the Second Congress of the International Association for the Scientific Study of Mental Deficiency*, Polish Medical Publishers, Warsaw.

Herman, A. (1981). *Guidance in Canadian Schools*, Dtselig, Calgary.

Holosko, M.J. (1987). A model for evaluating rehabilitation programmes: the case example of the St. John's job generation project. *National Consultation on Vocational Counselling* (in press).

Honzik, M.P., MacFarlane, J.W., and Allen, C. (1948). The stability of mental test performance between two and eighteen years, *Journal of Exceptional Education*, 17, 309−24.

Hughson, E.A. (1984). Behavioral and emotional aspects of training for adolescents and adults who are developmentally handicapped. In R.I. Brown (ed.), *Integrated Programmes for Developmentally Handicapped Adolescents and Adults*, A Series in Rehabilitation Education; Vol. 1, Croom Helm, London (Nichols, New York).

Hughson, E.A., and Brown, R.I. (1975). A bus training program for mentally retarded adults, *British Journal of Mental Subnormality*, XXI(2), 41, 79−83.

Hughson, E.A., and Brown, R.I. (1983). Some effects of verbal instruction on learning by developmentally handicapped adults, *Australia and New Zealand Journal of Developmental Disabilities*, 9(3), 107−16.

Hughson, E.A., Berien, V., and Brown, R.I. (1978). *Introductory Manual: Pre-Vocational Programme Packages*, Vocational and Rehabilitation Research Institute, Calgary, Canada.

Hussion, R. (1981). *Geriatric Psychology: A Behavioral Perspective*, Van Nostrand Reinhold, New York.

Hutchinson, D. (1983). *Work Preparation for the Handicapped*, Croom Helm, London.

Hutt, C., Hutt, S.J. and Ounstead, C. (1965). The behaviour of children with and without upper CNS lesions, *Behaviour*, 24(3−4), 246−68.

Huttenlocher, P.R. (1975). Synaptic and dendritic development and mental defect. In N.A. Buchwald and M.A.B. Brazier (eds), *Brain Mechanisms in Mental Retardation*, Academic Press, New York.

Itard, J.M.G. (1801). *The Wild Boy of Aveyron*. Translated by G. Humphrey and M. Humphrey (1932), Appleton Century, New York.

Jackson, R. (1984), Transition from school to adult life. In R.I. Brown (ed.), *Integrated Programmes for Handicapped Adolescents and Adults*, A Series in Rehabilitation Education, Vol. 1, Croom Helm, London (Nichols, New York).

Janicki, M.P., and Wisniewski, H.M. (1985). *Aging and Developmental Disabilities: Issues and Approaches*, Brookes, Baltimore, Maryland.

Jensen, A.R. (1970). A theory of primary and secondary familial mental retardation. In N.R. Ellis (ed.), *International Review of Research in Mental Retardation*, Vol. 4, Academic Press, New York.

Johnson, P.R. (1984), Interpersonal relationships: self-esteem, sexual intimacy, and life-long learning. In R.I. Brown (ed.), *Integrated Programmes for Handicapped Adolescents and Adults*, A Series in Rehabilitation Education, Vol. 1, Croom Helm, London (Nichols, New York).

Johnson, S.W., and Morasky, R.L. (1977). *Learning Disabilities*, Allyn & Bacon, Toronto.

Johnson-Martin, N., Jens, K.G., and Attermeier, S.M. (1986). *The Carolina Curriculum for Handicapped Infants and Infants at Risk*, P. Brookes, Baltimore, Maryland.

Jones, M. (1968), *Social Psychiatry in Practice: The Idea of a Therapeutic Community*, Penguin Books, Harmondsworth.

Jones, P.K., and Cregan, A. (1986). *Sign and Symbol, Communication for Mentally Handicapped People*, Croom Helm, London.

Jones, R.L., Lavine, K., and Shell, J. (1972). Blind children integrated in classrooms with sighted children: a sociometric study, *The New Outlook for the Blind*, 66, 75−80.

Kagan, J., (1984), *The Nature of the Child*, Basic Books, New York.

Kagan, J., and Moss, H.A. (1962). *From Birth to Maturity: a Study of the Psychological Development*, John Wiley, New York.

Kennett, K.R. (1986). Management and administration in rehabilitation: role of voluntary agencies and their boards. In R.I. Brown (ed.), *Management and Administration of Rehabilitation Programmes*, A Series in Rehabilitation Education, Vol. 2, Croom Helm, London (College Hill Press, San Diego, California).

Kinsbourne, M., and Caplan, P.J. (1979). *Children's Learning and Attention Problems*, Little, Brown & Co, Boston, Massachussetts.

Landino, J.E. (1979). Coding in the mentally retarded: Applications to learning and memory. Unpublished doctoral thesis, University of Calgary, Calgary, Alberta.

Lazar, I., and Darlington, R.B. (1978). *Lasting Effects after Preschool*, New York State College of Human Ecology, Cornell University.

Levine, S.P., Sharow, N., Gaudette, C., and Spector, S. (1984). *Recreation Experiences for the Severely Impaired or Non Ambulatory Child*, Charles C. Thomas, Springfield, Illinois.

Lewis, H. (1954). *Deprived Children*, Oxford Universiy Press, London.

Ley, P., and Spelman, M.S. (1965). Communication in an out-patient setting, *British Journal of Social and Clinical Psychology*, 4(2), 114−16.

Lorenz, K.E.Z. (1981). *The Foundations of Ethology*, Oxford University Press, Oxford.

Lovaas, O.I. (1966). A program for the establishment of speech in autistic children. In J.K. King (ed.), *Early Childhood Autism: Clinical, Educational and Social Aspects*, Pergamon, New York.

Luria, A.R. (1961). *The Role of Speech in the Regulation of Normal and Abnormal Behavior*, Pergamon, New York.

Marlett, N.J. (1971). *Adaptive Functioning Index*, Vocational and Rehabilitation Research Institute, Calgary (revised 1976).

Marlett, N.J. (1986). Impact of and alternates to corporate business models in rehabilitation. In R.I. Brown (ed.), *Management and Administration of Rehabilitation Programmes*, A Series in Rehabilitation Education, Vol. 2, Croom Helm, London (College Hill Press, San Diego, California).

Marlett, N.J. (1987). Disabled youth in transition: implications for social action approaches for rehabilitation counsellors, *National Consultation on Vocational Counselling* (in press).

Marlett, N.J., and Hughson, E.A. (1977). *Rehabilitation Programs Manual*, Vocational and Rehabilitation Research Institute, Calgary, Canada.

Martin, G., and Pear, J. (1983). *Behavior Modification: What It Is and How to Do It*, 2nd edn, Prentice Hall, Englewood Cliffs, New Jersey.

McCarthy, E.A. (1984). The possibility of integrated employment for Ireland's mentally handicapped workforce, *Journal of Practical Approaches to Developmental Handicap*, 8(2), 8−15.

McConkey, R.J., and Jeffree, D. (1981). *Making Toys for Handicapped Children. A Guide for Parents and Teachers*, Souvenir Press, London.

McDonald, J.R. (1982). *Human Service Planning, Accountability, Projection and Revision: a Needs Based Model Exemplified in Social Work Practice in Health Care*. Monograph, Faculty of Social Welfare, University of Calgary.

McFarland, D. (1981). *The Oxford Companion to Animal Behavior*, Oxford University Press, Oxford.

McKerracher, D.W. (1984). Progress in the assessment and prediction of vocational competence in the retarded. In R.I. Brown (ed.), *Integrated Programmes for Handicapped Adolescents and Adults*, A Series in Rehabilitation Education, Vol. 1, Croom Helm, London (Nichols, New York).

McKerracher, D.W., Brown, R.I., Marlett, N., and Zwirner, W.W. (1980). *A Study of the Utility of Assessment and Prediction Procedures in the Selection of Handicapped Persons for Industrial and Social Rehabilitation Programmes*. Final Report for Health and Welfare Canada (Grant No. 566-34-8), Vocational and Rehabilitation Research Institute, Calgary, Canada.

McLeod, J. (1985). An essay on computer-guided educational diagnosis. Paper presented at International Study Group on Special Education Needs Seminar, Copenhagen.

McLeod, M., and Brown, R.I. (1976). Verbal communication and the developmentally handicapped, *British Journal of Mental Subnormality*, **XXII**(1), 42, 26—34.

Meichenbaum, D. (1971a). The nature and modification of impulsive children. Paper presented at the Society for Research in Child Development, Minneapolis, Minnesota.

Meichenbaum, D. (1971b). Cognitive factors in behaviour modifications: modifying what people say to themselves. Paper presented at the 5th Annual Meeting of the Association for the Advancement of Behaviour Therapy, Washington, DC.

Meichenbaum, D., and Goodman, J. (1969). Reflection, impulsivity and verbal control of motor behaviour, *Child Development*, **40**, 785—97.

Meichenbaum, D., and Goodman, J. (1971) Training impulsive children to talk to themselves: a means of developing self control, *Journal of Abnormal Psychology*, **77**, 115—26.

Mendaglio, S. (1982), Burnout: an occupational hazard of the helping professions, *Journal of Practical Approaches to Developmental Handicap*, **6**(2/3), 34—38.

Mendaglio, S., and Swanson, D. (1986). Stress and burnout in rehabilitative settings. In R.I. Brown (ed.), *Management and Administration of Rehabilitation Programmes*, A Series in Rehabilitation Education, Vol. 2, Croom Helm, London (College Hill Press, San Diego, California).

Mitchell, D.R. (1986). A developmental systems approach to planning and evaluating services for persons with handicaps. In R.I. Brown (ed.), *Management and Administration of Rehabilitation Programmes*, A Series in Rehabilitation Education, Vol. 2, Croom Helm, London (College Hill Press, San Diego, California).

Mittler, P.J. (1970). *The Psychological Assessment of Physical and Mental Handicaps*, Methuen, London.

Mittler, P. (1977). *Research to Practice in Mental Retardation: Care and Intervention*, Vol. 1, University Park Press, Baltimore, Maryland.

Mittler, P. (1981). Strategies for manpower development in the 1980's, *Journal of Practical Approaches to Developmental Handicap*, **4**(3), 23—26.

Mosley, J.L. (1980). Selective attention of mildly mentally retarded and nonretarded individuals, *American Journal of Mental Deficiency*, **87**, 568—76.

Mosley, J.L. (1985). The high speed memory scanning task performance of mildly retarded and nonretarded individuals, *American Journal of Mental Deficiency*, **90**, 81—9.

Mundy, J.A. (1976). Conceptualization and program design, *Journal of Physical Education and Recreation*, 41—43.

Nash, J.B. (1953), *Philosophy of Recreation and Leisure*, William C. Brown, Dubuque, Iowa.

Negrin, S. (1983). Psychosocial aspects of aging and visual impairment, in R.T. Jose (ed.), *Understanding Low Vision*, American Foundation for the Blind, New York.

Neufeldt, A.H. (1986). Managing change in rehabilitation services. In R.I. Brown (ed.), *Management and Administration of Rehabilitation Programmes*, A Series in Rehabilitation Education, Vol. 2, Croom Helm, London (College Hill Press, San Diego, California).

Nihira, F.R., Shellhaus, M., and Leland, H. (1975). *Adaptive Behaviour Scales*, American Association for Mental Deficiency, Washington, DC.

Nirje, B. (1970). The normalization principle: implications and comments, *Journal of Mental Subnormality*, **16**, 62—70.

Norrie, B.I. (1970). Verbalisation and displacement behaviour. Unpublished M.Sc. thesis, University of Calgary, Calgary, Alberta.

O'Connor, N., and Tizard, J. (1956). *The Social Problem and Mental Deficiency*, Pergamon, London.

Olds, J. (1975). Unit recordings during Pavlovian conditioning. In N.A. Buchwald and M.A.B. Brazier (eds), *Brain Mechanisms in Mental Retardation*, Academic Press, New York.

Paine, S.C., Bellamy, G.T., and Wilcox, B. (1984). *Human Services that Work*, P.H. Brookes, Baltimore, Maryland.

Palmore, E. (1980). Social factors in aging. In E. Busse and D. Blazer (eds), *Handbook of Geriatric Psychiatry*, Van Nostrand Reinhold, New York.

Park, P. (ed.) (1986). The National People First Project, *The National Organizer*, National Institute on Mental Retardation, Toronto, Ontario.

Parmenter, T. (1983). Evaluation of rehabilitation programs for mentally retarded persons in Australia, *Journal of Practical Approaches to Developmental Handicap*, **7**(2), 3–6.

Parmenter, T.R. (1987). The importance of social networks to the quality of life of people with intellectual disabilities. In R.I. Brown (ed.), *Quality of Life and Rehabilitation*, A Series in Rehabilitation Education, Vol. 3, Croom Helm, London (in preparation).

Piaget, J. (1952a). *The Origins of Intelligence in Children*, International University Press, New York.

Piaget, J. (1952b). *Origin of Number Concepts in Children*, Routledge & Kegan Paul, London.

Piaget, J. and Inhelder, B. (1956). *The Child's Conception of Space*, Routledge & Kegan Paul, London.

Pond, D.A. (1961). Psychiatric aspects of epileptic and brain-damaged children, *British Medical Journal*, **2**, 1377–82, 1454–7.

Possberg, E., Beck-Ford, V., Brown, R.I., and Smith, N.E. (1979). *The Leisure Functioning Assessment*, Vocational and Rehabilitation Research Institute, Calgary, Alberta.

Prugh, D.G., Staug, E.M., Sands, H.H., Kirschbaum, R.M., and Lenihan, E.A. (1953). A study of the emotional reactions of children and families to hospitalization and illness, *American Journal of Orthopsychiatry*, **23**, 70–106.

Resnick, O. (1980). Studies on the effects of pre-natal protein malnutrition using the laboratory rat as a model, *Worcester Medical News*, **45**(3), 1–4.

Restak, R.M. (1979). *The Brain: The Last Frontier*, Doubleday, New York.

Rintala, D.H., Uhermohlen, D.M., Buck, E.L., Hanover, D., Alexander, J.L., Norris-Baker, C., Stephens, M.A.P., Willems, E.P., and Halstead, L.S. (1984). Self-observation and report technique (SORT). In A.S. Halpern and M.J. Fuhrer (eds), *Functional Assessment in Rehabilitation*, P.H. Brookes, Baltimore, Maryland.

Robins, L.N. (1966). *Deviant Children Grown Up*, Williams & Wilkins, Baltimore, Maryland.

Robinson, H.B., and Robinson, N.M.(1965). *The Mentally Retarded Child - A Psychological Approach*, McGraw-Hill, New York.

Robinson, H.B., and Robinson, N.M. (1970). Mental retardation. In P. H. Mussen (ed.), *Carmichael's Manual of Child Psychology*, Vol. 2, 3rd edn, Wiley, London.

Romig, D.A. (1978). Justice for our children, Lexington Books, Lexington, Massachusetts.

Rosen, M., Clarke, G.R., and Kivitz, M.S. (1977). *Habilitation of the Handicapped*, University Park Press, Baltimore, Maryland.

Rosenzweig, M.R., Bennett, E.L., and Diamond, M.C. (1972). Brain changes in response to experience, *Scientific American*, **226**(2), p. 22.

Rosenzweig, M.R., Bennett, E.L., and Diamond, M.C. (1976). Brain changes in response to experience. In M.R. Rosenzweig, E.L. Bennett and M.C. Diamond (eds), *Neuromechanisms of Learning and Memory*, MIT Press, Cambridge, Massachusetts.

Rutter, M. (1983). Developmental Neuropsychiatry, Guilford Press, New York.

Ryba, K.A., and Nolan, C.J.P. (1985). Computer learning systems for mentally retarded persons: interfacing theory with practice. In A.F. Ashman and R.S. Laura (eds), *The Education and Training of the Mentally Retarded*, Croom Helm, London.

Samuels, M. (1985). Personal communication. Calgary Society for Students with Learning Difficulties, Calgary, Alberta.

Sarason, S.B., and Doris, J. (1979). *Educational Handicap, Public Policy and Social History*, Free Press, New York.

Schaeffer, H.R. (1963). Some issues for research in the study of attachment behavior. In B. Fals (ed.), *Determinants of Infant Behavior*, Vol. 2, Methuen, London.

Schalock, R.L., Ross, B.C., and Ross, I. (1976). *Basic Skills Screening Test*, Mid-Nebraska Mental Retardation Services, Hastings, Nebraska.

Schulberg, H.C., and Baker, F. (1979). *Program Evaluation in the Health Fields*, Vol. II, Human Sciences Press, New York.

Segger, T.J., and Plecas, D.B. (1987). Developing life skills training for special clienteles: institutionalized offenders as a case in point, *National Consultation on Vocational Counselling* (in press).

Seguin, E. (1846). *Traitement Moral, Hygiene et Education des Idiots et des Autres Enfants Arrieres*, J.B. Baillière, Paris.

Seligman, M. (1979). *Strategies for Helping Parents of Exceptional Children*, Free Press, New York.

Sgroi, S.M. (1982). *Handbook of Clinical Intervention in Child Sexual Abuse*, Lexington Books, D.H. Heath, Lexington, Mass.

Shaw, R.C. (1984). *The Dellcrest Approach to the Management of Human Services: A Practical Guide for Board Members and Senior Managers*, The Dellcrest Children's Centre, Toronto, Ontario.

Skinner, B.F. (1957). *Verbal Behaviour*, Appleton-Century-Crofts, New York.

Sloan, W., and Stevens, H.A. (1976). *A Century of Concern*. A history of the American Association on Mental Deficiency, AAMR.

Sluckin, W. (1964). *Imprinting and Learning*, Methuen, London.

Smith, A. (1983a). Clinical psychological practice and principles of neuropsychological assessment. In E.C. Walker (ed.), *Handbook of Clinical Psychology Theory, Research and Practice*, Dow Jones-Irwin, Homewood, Illinois.

Smith, A. (1983b), Overview or underview, comment on Satz and Fletcher's 'Emergent trends in neuropsychology: an overview', *Journal of Consulting and Clinical Psychology*, **51**(5), 768–75.

Sokolov, A.N. (1969). Studies of speech mechanisms of thinking. In M. Cole and I. Moltzman (eds), *A Handbook of Contemporary Soviet Psychology*, Basic Books, London.

Sternberg, R.J. (1985). *Beyond IQ, A Triarchic Theory of Human Intelligence*, Cambridge University Press, New York.

Stott, D.H. (1977). Developing learning capacities in the retarded, *Journal of Practical Approaches to Developmental Handicap*, **1**(3), 19–31.

Strauss, A.A., and Lehtinen, L.C. (1960). *The Brain Injured Child*, Grune & Stratton, New York.

Sykes, S., and Smith, H. (1984). Preparing the mildly intellectually handicapped adolescent for employment and independent living: a research review. In R.I. Brown (ed.), *Integrated Programmes for Handicapped Adolescents and Adults*, A Series in Rehabilitation Education, Vol. 1, Croom Helm, London (Nichols, New York).

Tizard, J. (1974), Longitudinal and follow-up studies. In A.M. Clarke and A.D.B. Clarke (eds), *Mental Deficiency: The Changing Outlook*, 3rd edn, Methuen, London.

Toffler, A. (1980), *The Third Wave*, Bantam Books, New York.

Tredgold, A.F. (1949), *A Textbook of Mental Deficiency*, 7th edn reprinted (8th edn, 1952), Baillière, Tindall & Cox, London.

Tymchuk, A.J. (1974). *Behavior Modification with Children*, C.C. Thomas, Springfield, Illinois.

Tymchuk, A.J. (1979). *Parent and Family Therapy*, S.P. Medical and Scientific Books, New York.

Tzuriel, D., Samuels, M.T., and Feuerstein, R. (1987). Non-intellective factors in dynamic assessment. In R.M. Gupta and P. Coxhead (eds), *Cultural Diversity and Learning Efficiency*, Macmillan, London (in press).

Valverde, F. (1971). Rate and extent of recovery from dark rearing in the visual cortex of the mouse, *Brain Research*, **33**, 1–11.

Vandergoot, D., and Martin, E.W. (1986). Enhancing employment opportunities by involving business and industry in rehabilitation programs. In R.I. Brown (ed.), *Management and*

Administration of Rehabilitation Programmes, A Series in Rehabilitation Education, Vol. 2, Croom Helm, London (College Hill Press, San Diego, California).

Vernon, P.E. (1951). Recent investigations of intelligence and its measurement, *Eugenics Review*, **43**(3), 125–137.

Walsh, K.W. (1978), *Neuropsychology: A Clinical Approach*, Churchill Livingstone, New York.

Walsh, R.N., and Greenough, W.T. (1976). *Environments as Therapy for Brain Disfunction*, Plenum Press, New York.

Ward, J., Parmenter, T.J., Riches, V., and Hauritz, M. (1981). Predicting the outcome of a work preparation program, *Australian Journal of Developmental Disabilities*, **7**, 137–45.

Warren, B. (1984), *Using the Creative Arts in Therapy*, Croom Helm, London.

Weber, H. (1929). See Woodworth (1938), *Experimental Psychology*, Holt, New York.

Wehman, P. (1981). *Competitive Employment*, P.H. Brookes, Baltimore, Maryland.

Westwood, R. (1986), Conjoint evaluation as a programme development strategy. In R.I. Brown (ed.), *Management and Administration of Rehabilitation Programmes*, A Series in Rehabilitation Education, Vol. 2, Croom Helm, London (College Hill Press, San Diego, California).

Whelan, E., and Speake, B. (1979). *Learning to Cope*, Souvenir Press, Human Horizons Series, London.

Whelan, E., and Speake, B. (1981). *Getting to Work*, Souvenir Press, London.

Whelan, E., and Speake, B. (1984). Action research—working with adult training centres in Britain. In R.I. Brown (ed.), *Integrated Programmes for Handicapped Adolescents and Adults*, Vol. 1, Croom Helm, London (Nichols, New York).

Willer, B., and Guastaserro, J.R. (1987), Community living assessment for chronic mentally ill persons (in preparation).

Wolfensberger, W. (1967). Counselling the parents of the retarded. In A.A. Baumeister (ed.), *Mental Retardation*, Aldine, New York.

Wolfensberger, W. (1972). *Normalization: The Principle of Normalization in Human Services*, National Institute of Mental Retardation, Toronto.

Wolfensberger, W. (1983). Social role valorization: a proposed new term for the principle of normalization, *Mental Retardation*, **21**(6), 234–9.

Wolfensberger, W., and Glenn, L. (1975). *Programme Analysis of Service Systems Handbook*, 3rd edn, National Institute on Mental Retardation, Toronto.

Wolman, B. (1973). *Handbook of General Psychology*, Prentice Hall, Englewood Cliffs, New Jersey.

Woodward, M. (1960). Early experiences and later social responses of severely subnormal children, *British Journal of Medicine and Psychology*, **33**, 123–32.

Wortis, J. (ed.) (1981). *Mental Retardation and Developmental Disabilities*, Bruner/Mazel, New York.

Young, J., Rosati, R., and Vandergoot, D. (1986). Initiating a marketing strategy by assessing employer needs for rehabilitation services, *Journal of Rehabilitation*, April–June, 37–41.

Younghusband, E., Birchall, D., Davie, R., and Pringle, J.L. (1970), *Living with Handicap*, National Bureau for Cooperation in Child Care, London.

Zeaman, D., and House, B.J. (1963). The role of attention in retardate discrimination learning. In N.R. Ellis (ed.), *Handbook of Mental Deficiency*, McGraw-Hill, New York.

Zigler, E. (1966). Research on personality structure in the retardate. In Ellis, N.R. (ed.), *International Review of Research in Mental Retardation*, Vol. 1, Academic Press, London.

Author index

185

188

Subject index